武汉大学
优秀博士学位论文文库
编委会

主　任　李晓红

副主任　韩　进　舒红兵　李　斐

委　员（按姓氏笔画为序）

马费成　邓大松　边　专　刘正猷　刘耀林
杜青钢　李义天　李建成　何光存　陈　化
陈传夫　陈柏超　冻国栋　易　帆　罗以澄
周　翔　周叶中　周创兵　顾海良　徐礼华
郭齐勇　郭德银　黄从新　龚健雅　谢丹阳

武汉大学优秀博士学位论文文库

迷走神经诱发心房颤动的电生理和离子通道基础研究

The Basic Research of Electrophysiology and Ion Channel in Vagally Mediated Atrial Fibrillation

赵庆彦 著

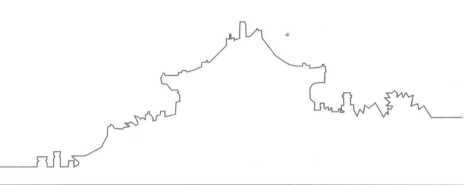

武汉大学出版社

图书在版编目(CIP)数据

迷走神经诱发心房颤动的电生理和离子通道基础研究/赵庆彦著.—武汉：武汉大学出版社,2014.1
武汉大学优秀博士学位论文文库
 ISBN 978-7-307-12347-2

Ⅰ.迷… Ⅱ.赵… Ⅲ.迷走神经—关系—心房纤颤—研究 Ⅳ.R541.7

中国版本图书馆 CIP 数据核字(2014)第 012614 号

责任编辑：黄汉平　　　责任校对：汪欣怡　　　版式设计：马　佳

出版发行：武汉大学出版社　（430072　武昌　珞珈山）
（电子邮件：cbs22@whu.edu.cn　网址：www.wdp.com.cn）
印刷：湖北恒泰印务有限公司
开本：720×1000　1/16　印张：6.5　字数：88 千字　插页：2
版次：2014 年 1 月第 1 版　　2014 年 1 月第 1 次印刷
ISBN 978-7-307-12347-2　　定价：18.00 元

版权所有，不得翻印；凡购我社的图书，如有质量问题，请与当地图书销售部门联系调换。

总　序

创新是一个民族进步的灵魂，也是中国未来发展的核心驱动力。研究生教育作为教育的最高层次，在培养创新人才中具有决定意义，是国家核心竞争力的重要支撑，是提升国家软实力的重要依托，也是国家综合国力和科学文化水平的重要标志。

武汉大学是一所崇尚学术、自由探索、追求卓越的大学。美丽的珞珈山水不仅可以诗意栖居，更可以陶冶性情、激发灵感。更为重要的是，这里名师荟萃、英才云集，一批又一批优秀学人在这里砥砺学术、传播真理、探索新知。一流的教育资源，先进的教育制度，为优秀博士学位论文的产生提供了肥沃的土壤和适宜的气候条件。

致力于建设高水平的研究型大学，武汉大学素来重视研究生培养，是我国首批成立有研究生院的大学之一，不仅为国家培育了一大批高层次拔尖创新人才，而且产出了一大批高水平科研成果。近年来，学校明确将"质量是生命线"和"创新是主旋律"作为指导研究生教育工作的基本方针，在稳定研究生教育规模的同时，不断推进和深化研究生教育教学改革，使学校的研究生教育质量和知名度不断提升。

博士研究生教育位于研究生教育的最顶端，博士研究生也是学校科学研究的重要力量。一大批优秀博士研究生，在他们学术创作最激情的时期，来到珞珈山下、东湖之滨。珞珈山的浑厚，奠定了他们学术研究的坚实基础；东湖水的灵动，激发了他们学术创新的无限灵感。在每一篇优秀博士学位论文的背后，都有博士研究生们刻苦钻研的身影，更有他们的导师的辛勤汗水。年轻的学者们，犹如在海边拾贝，面对知识与真理的浩瀚海洋，他们在导师的循循善诱下，细心找寻着、收集着一片片靓丽的贝壳，最终把它们连成一串串闪闪夺目的项链。阳光下的汗水，是他们砥砺创新的注脚；面向太阳的远方，是他们奔跑的方向；导师们的悉心指点，则是他们最值得依赖的臂膀！

博士学位论文是博士生学习活动和研究工作的主要成果，也是学校研究生教育质量的凝结，具有很强的学术性、创造性、规范性和专业性。博士学位论文是一个学者特别是年轻学者踏进学术之门的标志，很多博士学位论文开辟了学术领域的新思想、新观念、新视阈和新境界。

据统计，近几年我校博士研究生所发表的高质量论文占全校高水平论文的一半以上。至今，武汉大学已经培育出18篇"全国百篇优秀博士学位论文"，还有数十篇论文获"全国百篇优秀博士学位论文提名奖"，数百篇论文被评为"湖北省优秀博士学位论文"。优秀博士结出的累累硕果，无疑应该为我们好好珍藏，装入思想的宝库，供后学者慢慢汲取其养分，吸收其精华。编辑出版优秀博士学位论文文库，即是这一工作的具体表现。这项工作既是一种文化积累，又能助推这批青年学者更快地成长，更可以为后来者提供一种可资借鉴的范式亦或努力的方向，以鼓励他们勤于学习，善于思考，勇于创新，争取产生数量更多、创新性更强的博士学位论文。

武汉大学即将迎来双甲华诞，学校编辑出版该文库，不仅仅是为百廿武大增光添彩，更重要的是，当岁月无声地滑过120个春秋，当我们正大踏步地迈向前方时，我们有必要回首来时的路，我们有必要清晰地审视我们走过的每一个脚印。因为，铭记过去，才能开拓未来。武汉大学深厚的历史底蕴，不仅仅在于珞珈山的一草一木，也不仅仅在于屋檐上那一片片琉璃瓦，更在于珞珈山下的每一位学者和学生。而本文库收录的每一篇优秀博士学位论文，无疑又给珞珈山注入了新鲜的活力。不知不觉地，你看那珞珈山上的树木，仿佛又茂盛了许多！

李晓红

2013年10月于武昌珞珈山

摘 要

心房颤动(房颤)是临床上常见的快速房性心律失常,在人群中发病率较高,并发症较多,疗效欠佳。故需要更深刻地认识房颤的发生机制。房颤的发生机制复杂,可能与多种因素有关,但房颤的维持可能是通过电重构。房颤电重构是指房颤引起心房电生理功能的改变,是心房对房颤节律的病理生理性适应,包括动作电位时程(APD)及心房有效不应期(AERP)缩短,APD 及 AERP 的频率适应性降低,AERP 离散度(dAERP)和 APD 离散度(dAPD)增加。有研究认为自主神经尤其迷走神经在电重构中起重要作用,业已证实使用乙酰胆碱(Acetylcholine,Ach)或刺激迷走神经可引发房颤的发生;阻断迷走神经或去心房的迷走神经可以阻止或降低房颤的发生率。临床研究也显示,心脏结构正常的阵发性房颤患者在房颤起始和维持过程中,迷走神经起着重要作用,阵发性房颤患者在房颤发作前表现有自主神经张力的变化,而且阵发性房颤起始时间也影响了自主神经在阵发性房颤起始和终止时的张力,房颤复发与房颤复律后迷走神经张力占有势有关。

迷走神经对心房肌的影响是通过末梢释放 Ach 与心肌细胞膜上的胆碱能 M_2 受体结合,激活乙酰胆碱敏感钾通道电流(IK_{Ach}),促进 K^+ 外流使膜超极化。心房内神经支配的不均一可能是迷走神经刺激导致房颤的重要原因。有研究发现,随着 Ach 浓度的增加,优势频率在犬左右心房升高,但在左房占主导,转子数量比右房也多见,Kir3.4 和 Kir3.1mRNAs 在左房也比右房丰富。目前研究发现诱发房颤的大多数异位兴奋灶在肺静脉内,也可存在于上腔静脉、界嵴和左房后游离壁等。近来已经证明去迷走神经能提高环肺静脉消融治疗房颤的疗效,对阵发性和慢性房颤均有较高的成功率。

为了进一步探讨迷走神经张力在房颤复律前后对心房肌电生理的影响及异位兴奋灶诱发房颤与迷走神经的关系，本研究通过观察阻断迷走神经及刺激迷走神经对心房肌电生理的影响，以及 M_2 受体和 I_{KAch} 在心房及其相邻大静脉的分布情况，探讨迷走神经诱发房颤的离子机制。实验内容包括三部分。

第一部分，通过分析心率变异来反映迷走神经张力的变化，分析 AERP 反映心房电重构的变化，用动物实验模拟快速房率来观察阻断迷走神经对心房电重构变化的影响，并对其机制进行初步探讨。方法：用 8 只杂种犬自身随机对照，每只犬进行 3 次实验，共 24 次实验，分 3 组，每个实验组包括全部 8 只犬，采用频率为 800 次/min 快速刺激右心耳 7h。对照组：在心房快速刺激时和刺激终止后观察 AERP 及 dAERP 的变化，在心房快速刺激前和刺激终止后观察心率变异参数的变化；迷走神经阻断组：于快速刺激前 30min 静脉注入阿托品 0.04mg/kg 后 0.007mg/kg·h 维持，电生理监测同对照组；自主神经阻断组：于快速刺激前 30min 静注阿托品和普奈洛尔各 0.04mg/kg 和 0.2mg/kg，后阿托品以 0.007mg/kg·h 维持，普奈洛尔以 0.04mg/kg·h 维持，电生理监测同对照组。结果：①800 次/min 的快速心房刺激很快引起 AERP 缩短（$P<0.05$），dAERP 无明显变化。刺激终止后 AERP 恢复很快，dAERP 从 21 ± 5.3ms 升高到 40 ± 7.4ms（$P<0.05$）。②刺激终止后 HRV 参数明显升高（$P<0.05$）。③刺激前单用阿托品，AERP 从 128 ± 12ms 升高到 135 ± 12ms（$P>0.05$），dAERP 无明显变化，快速刺激仍能引起 AERP 缩短，刺激终止后 dAERP 升高不明显。③刺激前联用阿托品和普奈洛尔，AERP 从 127 ± 12ms 升高到 142 ± 14ms（$P<0.05$），dAERP 无明显变化，快速刺激仍能引起 AERP 缩短，刺激终止后 dAERP 升高不明显。

本部分实验结论：阻断迷走神经不能阻止电重构的发生，但迷走神经张力变化与 dAERP 有密切关系，基础状态下迷走神经张力对 dAERP 没有明显影响，而迷走神经高张力才对 dAERP 有明显升高作用，且迷走神经与交感神经对 AERP 有协同作用。

第二部分，通过迷走神经刺激（VS）观察犬在体情况下心房肌不同部位 APD 的变化，并观察胺碘酮对 VS 诱发房颤的影响，探讨其诱发房颤的机制。方法：成年杂种犬 10 只，麻醉后经胸骨行正中开胸术，切开心包暴露心脏。制备特制的电极固定在心房肌外膜，包括右心耳、高位右心房、低位右心房、左心耳、高位左心房、低位左心房。共计录 6 个不同部位的 APD。10 只犬采用自身对照。其中每只犬在开胸的同时，分离左右颈部迷走神经干，切断双侧迷走神经（0.2mg/kg 普奈洛尔静注阻断交感神经）。然后刺激迷走神经干远端（频率 20Hz，0.2ms 波宽，10V 电压，作为 VS_1）；停止 VS_1，待心房 MAP 和心率完全恢复后，然后用电生理刺激仪，以刺激频率 20Hz 和 0.2ms 的刺激波宽，30V 的电压刺激迷走神经干远端（作为 VS_2）；停止 VS_2，待心房 MAP 和心率完全恢复后，钳夹阻断升主动脉 2~3s，同时于主动脉根部注入 Ach 20~60μmol/L，使 Ach 灌注到冠状动脉，灌注剂量以引起心率减慢大致等同 VS_1；待心房 MAP 和心率完全恢复后，静脉注入胺碘酮 1mg/kg，5 分钟后再次 VS_1。其中在 VS_1 前、VS_1 时、VS_2 时、灌注 Ach 时和 VS_1+胺碘酮时，同时观察心房肌 APD 变化，并在右心耳给一电刺激，观察诱发房颤的情况。将每只犬在基础状态下的 MAP 记录作为对照组；每只犬在 VS_1 状态下完成的 MAP 记录作为 VS_1 组；每只犬在 VS_2 状态下完成的 MAP 记录作为 VS_2 组；每只犬在灌注 Ach 状态下完成的 MAP 记录作为 Ach 灌注组；每只犬在 VS_1+胺碘酮状态下完成的 MAP 记录作为 VS_1+胺碘酮组。五组均于记录 MAP 图形时，同步记录心电图。结果：对照组有 2 例诱发房早，无一例诱发出房颤；VS_1 组 7 例诱发房颤；VS_2 组 8 例诱发房颤；Ach 灌注组 6 例诱发房颤；VS_1+胺碘酮组诱发 2 例房颤。VS_1、VS_2 和 Ach 灌注明显缩短 APD_{50}、APD_{90}，其中心耳缩短最明显（APD_{50} 从 72±5ms 到 19±4ms，APD_{90} 从 136±7ms 到 43±5ms，$P<0.001$）；VS_1 和 Ach 灌注组都明显升高心房肌 APD_{90} 离散（VS_1：5±3ms 比 11±5ms，7±5ms 比 19±7ms，$P<0.01$），而 VS_2 与对照组相比，dAPD 没有明显差异。胺碘酮组诱发房颤的比率比 VS 组有明显降低（$P<0.05$）。胺碘酮组与对照组相比，APD 也明显

3

缩短。

本部分实验结论：VS 的强度与 dAPD 有明显关系，VS 诱发房颤的基础主要是 APD 缩短，VS 和 Ach 灌注都易诱发房颤的发生，并且对心耳 APD 的影响较大，即 VS 或 Ach 灌注对心耳的 APD 缩短更明显。胺碘酮能有效地降低迷走神经刺激对 APD 的影响及其诱发房颤的几率。

第三部分，通过对胆碱能 M_2 和 I_{KAch} 受体在犬心房及其相邻大静脉的分布研究，及胺碘酮对 I_{KAch} 的影响，提供和探讨迷走神经诱发心房内折返和房颤的分子和离子通道基础。方法：30 只犬通过迷走神经刺激（刺激频率 20Hz 和 0.2ms 的刺激波宽，10~30V 的电压），根据诱发房颤情况分为房颤组和对照组。迷走神经刺激后，取出心脏，分离出左右心耳、左右心房、肺静脉和上腔静脉，分别用 Western 印记法和膜片钳全细胞法分析 M_2 受体和 $I_{K,Ach}$ 在心耳、心房、肺静脉和上腔静脉的分布，并应用胺碘酮后观察对 $I_{K,Ach}$ 的变化。结果：30 只犬迷走神经刺激有 18 只诱发出房颤，作为房颤组；12 只未诱发出房颤，作为对照组。房颤组：M_2 受体蛋白和 I_{KAch} 在左心耳、右心耳和左心房的分布明显高于右心房、肺静脉和上腔静脉（M_2 受体：0.66 ± 0.08，0.67 ± 0.08 and 0.51 ± 0.06 vs 0.35 ± 0.04，0.33 ± 0.04 and 0.32 ± 0.03 $P < 0.05$；$I_{K,Ach}$：$20.36 \pm 0.91(n=6)$、$21.23 \pm 0.95(n=6)$、$14.17 \pm 0.65(n=5)$ vs $10.34 \pm 0.62(n=6)$、$8.24 \pm 0.45(n=6)$、$7.65 \pm 0.42(n=7)$ pA/pF $P < 0.05$），而且左右心耳的分布也明显比左心房高，$P < 0.05$；对照组：M_2 受体蛋白和 I_{KAch} 在左心耳、右心耳和左心房的分布也明显高于右心房、肺静脉和上腔静脉（M_2 受体：0.52 ± 0.06，0.53 ± 0.06 and 0.50 ± 0.05 vs 0.34 ± 0.04，0.31 ± 0.03 and 0.32 ± 0.03. $P < 0.05$；I_{KAch}：$16.27 \pm 0.87(n=6)$、$16.75 \pm 0.82(n=6)$、$14.78 \pm 0.63(n=5)$ vs $10.65 \pm 0.48(n=6)$、$8.35 \pm 0.41(n=6)$、$7.34 \pm 0.37(n=7)$ pA/pF $P < 0.05$），但左右心耳和左心房的分布没有明显差异。I_{KAch} 都表现出强的内向整流性，在超极化有逐渐升高的内向电流，而在去极化表现快速衰减的外向电流，在房颤组，2mmol/L 胺碘酮阻断后，I_{KAch} 强度均明显减小，但左右心耳的 I_{KAch}

强度仍比左右心房、肺静脉和上腔静脉大，左右心房的电流密度没有明显差异(6.86 ± 0.51 vs 6.67 ± 0.59, $P<0.05$)。房颤组和对照组相比，左心耳、右心耳的 M_2 受体和 I_{KAch} 在房颤组也比对照组高。

  本部分实验结论：M_2 受体蛋白和 I_{KAch} 在心房肌的分布是不均一的，这种不均一可能是迷走神经刺激诱发折返和房颤的分子基础。心耳的分布明显高于其他部位，心耳可能在迷走神经诱发房颤中有重要作用。而肺静脉和上腔静脉对迷走性房颤的作用较小。胺碘酮可以阻断 I_{KAch} 并减少左右心房 I_{KAch} 大小的差异，此可能是其治疗胆碱能房颤的机制。

关键词：迷走神经 心房颤动 电生理 电重构 单项动作电位 M_2 受体 乙酰胆碱敏感钾通道

Abstract

Atrial fibrillation(AF) is a frequent atrial arrhythmia in clinic. The disease incidence is high and the success rate to cardioversion is low. Therefore, to study the mechanism of AF is imperative. The mechanism of AF perhaps has relation with multi-factors, however, atrial eletrical remodeling (AER) may plays an important role in the maintenance of AF. AER is a change in atrial electrophysiology, including the shorten of action potential duration (APD) and atrial effective refractory period (AERP), the increase of dispersion of APD and AERP, and the loss of the physiological rate adaptation of the AERP. Studies suggested the autonomic nervous system (ANS), especially the vagus play an important role. It has been well established that Acetylcholine (Ach) administration and vagal nerve stimulation can induce the pathogenesis of AF. Catheter ablation of the cardiac parasympathetic nerves abolishes vagally-mediated AF.

Clinical observations suggest that the parasympathetic nervous system, at least in some patients with paroxysmal AF and structurally normal hearts, may play a role in the initiation and/or maintenance of AF. The occurrence of AF depends on variations of the autonomic tone, with a primary increase in adrenergic tone followed by an abrupt shift toward vagal predominance.

Parasympathetic stimulation causes release of acetylcholine (Ach) from the vagus nerve in the atria. Ach after binding with the M_2 muscarinic receptors in the atrial cell membrane causes activation of the inhibitory G proteins which activates the G-protein-gated inward rectifier K^+

channels. The heterogeneous innervation of the atria by vagus nerve terminal can cause dispersion and AF. Sarmast et al. demonstrated in the isolated sheep atrium that a greater abundance of Kir3.x channels and higher $I_{K,Ach}$ density in left atrium(LA) than right atrium(RA) myocytes result in greater Ach-induced speeding-up of rotors in the LA than in the RA. the role of vagal denervation in enhancing long-term benefits from circumferential pulmonary vein (PV) ablation.

To further investigate the effect of vagal tone on atrium before and after AF cardioversion. , the present study was conducted to observe the effect of vagus in atrial electrophysiology by blockage and stimulation, and differential densities of M_2 receptor and I_{KAch} in atrium, atrial appendage, PV and super vena cava (SVC). This study included three parts.

The first part was to characterize the effect of vagus on AER as well as define possible mechanisms of the phenomenon. 8 dogs, were used in the study for three consecutive protocol. At first, dogs were subjected to atrial pacing at 800ppm for 7 hours, and AERP was measured at every hour at 6 sites in the status of non-pacing. Subsequently, pacing was stopped and the electrophysiological study was repeated each hour for 7 hours. Time-domain parameters of heart rate variability (HRV) were also computed 1 hour before pacing as well as each hour after non-pacing. Secondly, program was performed after two weeks following first one, and 0.04mg/kg of atropine was intravenously administration 30 min before pacing, and then 0.007mg/kg was added at each hour. The procedure of second protocol was nearly same as the first one, while parameters of HRV were not evaluated. Finally, dogs were subjected to third protocol at two weeks after completion of second one. The procedure of third protocol was nearly same as the second one except 0.2mg/kg of propranolol was intravenously administration 30 min before pacing, and 0.04mg/kg was added at each hour. The dispersion of AERP (dAERP) was calculated maximum AERP minus minimum AERP. The data showed that there was a prompt decrease in AERP as the result of pacing ($P<0.05$), but dAERP didn't change significantly. The AERP recovered quickly, and dAERP increased from 21 ± 5.3ms to 40 ± 7.4ms ($P<0.05$) after cessation of pacing. At the same time, the parameters of HRV increased ($P<0.05$) after cessation of pacing. The AERP increased from 128 ± 12ms to 135 ± 12ms and from 127 ± 12ms to 142 ± 14ms ($P<0.05$) after vagal and autonomic blockade. However, AERP decreased during pacing ($P<0.05$) in the condition of vagal or autonomic blockade, but dAERP did not change significantly during and after pacing. Conclusions: These results suggest that vagal and autonomic blockade can not prevent AER, but a high vagal tone is associated with a high dAERP during recovery from AER, indicating that Vagus and sympathetic have a synergism on the refractory period.

The aim of the second study was to investigate the electrophysiological effect of vagal stimulation (VS), Ach administration and amiodarone on atrial myocardium in vivo and to discuss the mechanisms of AF. After a median sternotomy, the heart was exposed in a pericardial cradle. With the monophasic action potential (MAP) recording technique, right atrial appendage (RAA), high RA, low RA, left atrial appendage (LAA), high LA, and low LA were recorded by custom-built electrode probes applied to the epicardial atrial surface in dogs. After cervical vagosympathetic cut (0.2mg/kg of propranolol was intravenously administration), VS_1, VS_2, Ach perfusion and VS_1 + amiodarone were administrated respectively. At the same time, MAP, dispersion of action potential duration (dAPD) and AF were investigated. During VS_1, VS_2, and Ach perfusion, AF was evoked easily. APD_{50} and APD_{90} abbreviated significantly during VS as well as during Ach perfusion (RAA, APD_{50} from 72 ± 5ms to 19 ± 4ms, APD_{90} from 136 ± 7ms to 43 ± 5ms, $P<0.001$). However, compared with the data in VS and Ach perfusion groups, APD_{50} and APD_{90} were prolonged during VS_1 + amiodarone. During VS_1 and Ach perfusion, dAPD was increased significantly in

APD_{90} (VS_1: APD_{50}, from 5 ± 3ms to 11 ± 5ms, APD_{90}, from 7 ± 5ms to 19 ± 7ms, and Ach perfusion: APD_{90}, from 7 ± 5ms to 15 ± 7ms, $P < 0.01$), but there was no significant difference in VS_2 and VS_1 + amiodarone group. Conclusions: The intensity of vagus has highly relationship with dAPD. Decreased APD is the base in initiation of cholinergic AF by VS. Reduce the effect of VS on APD and dAPD is the mechanism for amiodarone to therapy vagally-mediated AF.

The purpose of the third part was to investigate the distribution of M_2 receptor subtyps and acetylcholine activated K^+ current ($I_{K,Ach}$) in PV, SVC, LAA, RAA, RA and LA, and discuss the molecular basis of cholinergic AF. Method: Thirty dogs abdomenly anesthetized with pentobarbital sodium. After VS, thirty dogs were divided AF group (AF could be induced) and control group (AF could not be induced). Western-blot and patch clamp were used to determin M_2 receptor and $I_{K,Ach}$ in LAA, RAA, LA, RA, PV and SVC. During VS, AF was induced in 18 dogs, but not induced in 12 dogs. In control group, the densities of M_2 receptor and $I_{K,Ach}$ in LAA, RAA and LA were higher than that in RA, PV and SVC (M_2 receptor: 0.52 ± 0.06, 0.53 ± 0.06 and 0.50 ± 0.05 vs 0.34 ± 0.04, 0.31 ± 0.03 and 0.32 ± 0.03. $P < 0.05$; I_{KAch}: $16.27 \pm 0.87 (n=6)$、$16.75 \pm 0.82 (n=6)$、$14.78 \pm 0.63 (n=5)$ vs $10.65 \pm 0.48 (n=6)$、$8.35 \pm 0.41 (n=6)$、$7.34 \pm 0.37 (n=7)$ pA/pF $P < 0.05$). However, there was no significant difference in LAA, RAA and LA. In AF group, The densities of M_2 receptor and $I_{K,Ach}$ in LAA, RAA and LA were higher than that in RA, PV and SVC (M_2 receptor: 0.66 ± 0.08, 0.67 ± 0.08 and 0.51 ± 0.06 vs 0.35 ± 0.04, 0.33 ± 0.04 and 0.32 ± 0.03 $P < 0.05$; $I_{K,Ach}$: $20.36 \pm 0.91 (n=6)$、$21.23 \pm 0.95 (n=6)$、$14.17 \pm 0.65 (n=5)$ vs $10.34 \pm 0.62 (n=6)$、$8.24 \pm 0.45 (n=6)$、$7.65 \pm 0.42 (n=7)$ pA/pF $P < 0.05$). Furthermore, the densities of the M_2 and $I_{K,Ach}$ in LAA and RAA were higher than that in LA. $I_{K,Ach}$ demonstrated strong inward rectification with increasing inward currents during hyperpolarizing voltage steps and rapidly decaying outward currents during depolarization. In AF group, After amiodarone administration, densities of $I_{K,Ach}$ in LA and RA were not difference, but densities of $I_{K,Ach}$ were also less in atrium than in atrial appendage. Compared with the data in control group, the densities of M_2 receptor and $I_{K,Ach}$ in LAA, RAA were higher in AF group. There was no significant difference in LA, RA, PV and SVC between control group and AF group. Conclusions: Densities of the M_2 receptor and $I_{K,Ach}$ are higher in atrial appendage than other sites. Atrial appendage perhaps play an important role in initiation of cholinergic AF. However, PV and SVC less often play an important role in vagotonic paroxysmal AF. Reduced dispersion of $I_{K,Ach}$ is the mechanism for amiodarone to therapy AF.

Key wards: vagal nerve, atrial fibrillation, Electrophysiology, eletrical remodeling, monophasic action potential, M_2 receptor subtype, acetylcholine activated K^+ current

目 录

引言 ··· 1

第1章 迷走神经对心房肌电重构影响的实验研究 ············ 4
材料与方法 ·· 4
    1. 主要材料 ··· 4
    2. 实验对象 ··· 5
    3. 实验方法 ··· 5
    4. 统计学分析 ··· 6
结果 ·· 8
    1. 电生理变化 ··· 8
    2. 心率变异变化 ·· 8
讨论 ·· 12
结论 ·· 14

第2章 迷走神经刺激和乙酰胆碱灌注对心房肌电生理的影响 ·· 15
材料与方法 ··· 15
    1. 主要材料 ·· 15
    2. 实验对象 ·· 16
    3. 实验方法 ·· 16
结果 ·· 18
    1. 各组中诱发房早、房颤的情况 ······························ 18

  2. 各组心外膜 MAP 时程长短的变化 ………………………… 18
  3. 各组心外膜 dAPD 的变化 …………………………………… 18
 讨论 ………………………………………………………………… 22
 结论 ………………………………………………………………… 24

第3章 胆碱能 M_2 受体和乙酰胆碱敏感钾通道在心房肌及其相邻大静脉的分布研究 ……………… 25

 材料与方法 ………………………………………………………… 25
  1. 主要材料 ……………………………………………………… 25
  2. 实验对象 ……………………………………………………… 27
  3. 实验方法 ……………………………………………………… 27
  4. 统计学处理 …………………………………………………… 31
 结果 ………………………………………………………………… 32
  1. Western-blot 分析结果 ……………………………………… 32
  2. I_{KAch} 的分布特点 …………………………………………… 34
 讨论 ………………………………………………………………… 39
 结论 ………………………………………………………………… 42

第4章 综述：迷走神经与心房颤动 …………………………… 43

 1. 心房的迷走神经支配 …………………………………………… 43
 2. 迷走神经与房颤的关系 ………………………………………… 44
 3. 迷走神经对心房颤动电重构的影响 …………………………… 46
 4. 迷走神经对心房颤动影响的离子通道基础 …………………… 50
 5. 心脏迷走神经消融在房颤中的作用 …………………………… 54

参考文献 ……………………………………………………………… 59

后记 …………………………………………………………………… 84

引 言

心房颤动（房颤）是临床最常见的持续性心律失常，一般人群中房颤的患病率大概为0.5%，并且随年龄增长其发生率也随之升高[1]。房颤已经成为影响公众健康的主要疾病之一，因此也是目前心血管领域研究的热点。关于房颤的发生机制主要涉及两个基本方面，其一是房颤的触发因素（trigger），触发因素是多种多样的，包括异位兴奋灶、交感或副交感神经刺激、房性早搏或心动过速和急性心房牵拉等，目前发现大多数异位兴奋灶在肺静脉内，也可存在上腔静脉、界嵴和左房后游离壁等[2~9]。其二是房颤维持的基质（substrate），心房具有发生房颤的基质是房颤发作和维持的必要条件，以心房有效不应期的缩短和心房扩张为特征的电重构和解剖重构是房颤持续的基质，重构变化可能有利于形成多重折返子波。此外，还与心房有效不应期的离散度增加和包括局部阻滞、传导减慢和心肌束的分隔等传导的不均一性增加有关[10~14]。

刺激迷走神经可诱发房颤的发生；阻断迷走神经或去心房的迷走神经可以阻止或降低房颤的发生[15,16]。心脏结构正常的阵发性房颤患者，迷走神经对房颤起始和维持都起重要作用[17~19]，阵发性房颤患者在房颤发作前表现有自主神经张力的变化，即发作前数分钟先表现为交感神经张力的升高，随后出现迷走神经张力占优势[20,21]，而且阵发性房颤起始时间也影响了自主神经在阵发性房颤起始和终止时的张力[22]。Bertaglia等对25例持续性房颤病人进行电转复后观察其心率变异性的变化，48h内房颤再复发病人比没有复发病人的LLF/HF的比率明显低，他认为房颤在48h内复发与房颤复律后迷走神经张力占优势有关[23]。

近来报道联合消融肺静脉的异位兴奋灶和迷走神经比单独消融异位兴奋灶后房颤的复发率明显降低；基础研究也发现对犬的心房脂肪垫消融可以阻止迷走神经介导房颤的诱发[24]。但Oral等[25]对阵发性房颤病人进行肺静脉电隔离消融，依据病史分为迷走神经性房颤、肾上腺能房颤和随机发生的房颤，却发现肺静脉电隔离对迷走神经性房颤的治疗效果最低。Razavi[26]在对犬的肺静脉电隔离消融后发现左房的心房有效不应期（AERP）对迷走神经刺激的反应性下降，房颤的易损性也明显降低。结果提示对肺静脉电隔离和去迷走神经消融治疗房颤，房颤的复发率下降可能不是肺静脉去迷走神经后的直接原因，而是因为肺静脉电隔离和去迷走神经后，导致迷走神经刺激对心房和心耳的影响下降的原因。

迷走神经对心房肌的影响是通过末梢释放乙酰胆碱（Ach）与心肌细胞膜上的胆碱能 M_2 受体结合，激活 Ach 敏感钾通道电流（IK_{Ach}）。心房内神经支配的不均一可能是迷走神经刺激导致房颤的重要原因，Sarmast 等[27]采用光学标测和双极记录观察绵羊诱发房颤的情况，其中优势频率和动态定量分别由光电信号和相位电影来判断，发现随着 Ach 浓度的增加，优势频率在左右心房升高，但在左房占主导，转子数量比右房也多见，Kir3.4 和 Kir3.1mRNAs 在左房也比右房丰富。Lomax 等[28]实验证实鼠的左房心肌细胞比右房心肌细胞有更高的外向快速延迟整流和内向整流钾电流。电压和时间依赖钾电流的梯度导致在左房的 APD 比右房更短。电压和时间依赖性电流之间的相互作用、I_{KAch} 表现的不同水平和神经末梢空间分布不同改变 AERP，进而引起折返。但是 Lomax 等[29]在另一次实验发现成鼠右房心肌的 I_{KAch} 却明显高于左房，与 K_{Ach} 是否被毒蕈碱或 A_1 受体激动剂激动无关。

由此可见，迷走神经诱发心房内折返和房颤的机制还不明确，而且去迷走神经治疗房颤的机制也有不同的认识。有研究发现诱发房颤的大多数异位兴奋灶在肺静脉内，也可存在上腔静脉、界嵴和左房后游离壁等。为了进一步探讨迷走神经张力在房颤复律前后对心房肌电生理的影响及异位兴奋灶诱发房颤与迷走神经的关系，本

引 言

研究旨在观察快速心房刺激时,阻断迷走神经前后对心房肌电重构的影响,探讨迷走神经诱发房颤的电生理机制;并进一步研究 M_2 受体和 I_{KAch} 在心房肌及其相邻大静脉的分布情况,为认识迷走神经诱发房颤的机制提供部分分子和离子通道改变的实验数据。

第1章 迷走神经对心房肌电重构影响的实验研究

近年来有学者在慢性房颤动物模型中研究房颤的电生理机制时发现电重构现象[1,2]。电重构现象表现为心房有效不应期（AERP）和动作电位时程缩短等，电重构的机制目前不十分明了，有研究认为自主神经尤其迷走神经在电重构中起重要作用，临床观察显示副交感神经张力升高是阵发性房颤发生的原因[3-7]，迷走神经张力增加是房颤复律后再发的因素。但迷走神经在房颤复律前后对心房肌电生理的作用还不明了。此研究我们通过分析心率变异性（HRV）反映迷走神经的变化，分析 AERP 反映心房电重构的变化来观察阻断迷走神经对电重构的影响。

材料与方法

1. 主要材料

1.1 主要仪器

心率变异心电分析系统	美国 Mars3000 型
32 道心电生理监测仪	四川锦江产 LEAD-2000B 型
程序快速刺激仪	苏州产 DF-5A 型
C 臂 X 光机	荷兰 Philip 公司
6F 四极电极导管	Cordis 公司
电子秤	瑞典 AE200S

1.2 主要试剂

肝素针剂	广东天普生化公司

阿托品针剂	上海第一生化药业有限公司
普奈洛尔针剂	常州四药制药有限公司
戊巴比妥钠	上海三爱思试剂公司

2. 实验对象

由武汉大学人民医院动物房提供成年杂种犬 8 只，雌雄不拘，体重 19~26kg。

3. 实验方法

3.1 动物准备

以 30mg/kg 剂量的戊巴比妥钠腹腔麻醉（根据动物反应每 30~60min 静脉追加戊巴比妥钠 50mg），气管插管（实验期间如呼吸不稳人工通气），麻醉后右侧颈部备皮（12cm×12cm），充分暴露颈内静脉以利插管，胸壁备皮（20cm×20cm）清洁皮肤以贴电极。固定手术床，常规消毒铺巾。

3.2 心率变异监测及分析指标

采用心电分析系统及其心率变异分析软件，逐个识别标记 R 波，删除早搏和伪差。所有犬均于上午 8~9 时静脉插管后记录。刺激前，窦性心律时记录 1 h，刺激终止后恢复为窦性心律时再记录 7 h。有效记录时间 8~9 h。

分析指标：

① SDNNms：单位时间内连续的窦性 RR 间期标准差；

② SDANNms：单位时间内连续 5 min 窦性 RR 间期均数的标准差；

③ SDNNindexms：单位时间内连续 5 min 窦性 RR 间期标准差的均数；

④ rMSSDms：单位时间内连续窦性 RR 间期差的均方根；

⑤ PNN_{50}：单位时间内相临 RR 间期差值大于 50 ms 占的百分比。

3.3 导管放置与电生理检查

在 X 线透视下将 3 根 6F 四极电极导管经右侧股静脉分别置于高位右房、右房侧壁及低位右房，2 根 6F 四极导管经右颈内静脉分别置于右心耳、冠状静脉窦，静脉注入肝素 1000IU。连接 32 道心电生理监测仪，共计录 5 个不同部位 AERP。刺激前，先测量基础状态 AERP，测量 AERP 采用 S_1S_2 程序刺激法，首先进行 8 次 S_1S_1 刺激，S_1S_1 为 300ms，输出脉宽 2ms，强度为 2 倍舒张阈强度，然后在心房舒张晚期进行一次程序早搏 S_2 刺激，每次提前 5ms。程序早搏刺激未引起心房应激的最长 S_1S_2 间期为 AERP，其中最大 AERP 值与最小 AERP 值的差值为 dAERP。然后开始快速刺激，刺激部位在右心耳（S_1S_2 程序刺激和快速刺激仪均为苏州产 DF-5A 型），频率为 800 次/min。快速刺激共 7h，每 h 中断一次测量 AERP，刺激终止后同样每 h 测量一次 AERP，7 h 后结束。

3.4 阻断神经与分组

8 只犬自身对照，每只犬进行 3 次实验，共 24 次实验，分 3 组，每个实验组包括全部 8 只犬（图 1-1）。

①对照组：完成上述各项检查（包括 HRV 检测、基础状态及快速刺激前后的电生理检查）。

②迷走神经阻断组：于快速刺激前 30 min 静脉注入（简称静注）阿托品 0.04mg/kg 后 0.007mg/kg·h 维持，电生理监测同对照组。

③自主神经阻断组：于快速刺激前 30 min 静注阿托品和普奈洛尔各 0.04mg/kg 和 0.2mg/kg，后阿托品以 0.007mg/kg·h 维持，普奈洛尔以 0.04mg/kg·h 维持（此剂量可起完全阻断作用[8]），电生理监测同对照组。

实验后拔除导管，纱布包扎伤口，肌注青霉素 240 万 IU，预防感染。麻醉恢复后送回动物房，2 周后重复实验。

4. 统计学分析

数据以均数 ± 标准差（$\bar{x} \pm s$）表示，用 t 检验和方差分析进行统计学处理，以 $P<0.05$ 为差异有显著性。

第1章 迷走神经对心房肌电重构影响的实验研究

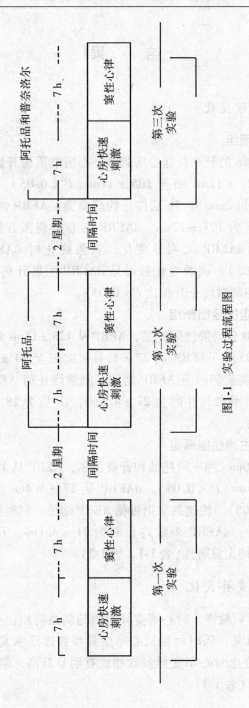

图1-1 实验过程流程图

结　果

1. 电生理变化

1.1 对照组

800次/min的频率快速心房刺激，心房电重构开始较快，第1 h AERP从 127 ± 12 ms 缩至 105 ± 11 ms($P<0.05$)，之后的6 h AERP平均缩短2ms/h，7h后停止快速刺激，AERP恢复较快，1h后AERP恢复为 107 ± 12 ms。dAERP在心房刺激开始时为 28 ± 5.6 ms，之后dAERP无明显变化，刺激终止时dAERP为 21 ± 5.3 ms($P>0.05$)。刺激终止后可见dAERP明显升高，7h后达到 40 ± 7.4 ms(与刺激终止时相比 $P<0.05$)。

1.2 迷走神经阻断组

刺激前30分钟静注阿托品，AERP从 128 ± 12 ms 延长至 135 ± 12 ms($P>0.05$)，dAERP从 27 ± 5.4 ms 缩短至 24 ± 4.1 ms($P>0.05$)。快速刺激仍可见AERP缩短，刺激终止时AERP为 106 ± 10 ms。dAERP刺激终止时为 21 ± 4.1 ms，7h后为 28 ± 5.1 ms，差异均无显著性。

1.3 自主神经阻断组

刺激前30min静注阿托品和普奈洛尔，AERP从 127 ± 12 ms 延长至 142 ± 14 ms($P<0.05$)，dAERP从 27 ± 5.4 ms 缩短至 24 ± 4.1 ms($P>0.05$)。快速刺激仍可见AERP缩短，刺激终止时AERP为 109 ± 10 ms。dAERP刺激终止时为 21 ± 4.1 ms，7h后为 28 ± 5.1 ms，差异均无显著性(表1-1，表1-2)。

2. 心率变异变化

对照组：刺激终止时心率变异参数与刺激前相比有下降趋势，但无统计学意义，随时间延长心率变异参数逐渐恢复，刺激终止7h后与刺激终止时心率变异参数相比有明显升高，但与刺激前相比无明显差异(表1-3)。

表 1-1 各组 AERP 在心房快速刺激下的变化（$\bar{x} \pm s$, ms）

组别	n	刺激前	刺激时						
			1h	2h	3h	4h	5h	6h	7h
对照组	8	127±12	105±11△	103±10△	103±11△	101±10△	98±10△	97±10△	96±10△
迷走神经阻断组	8	135±12	116±12△	115±12△	113±12△	113±11△	111±11△	108±10△	106±10△
自主神经阻断组	8	142±14*	121±12△	120±12△	117±12△	116±11△	115±11△	112±10△	109±10△

组别	n	刺激前	刺激终止后						
			1h	2h	3h	4h	5h	6h	7h
对照组	8	127±12	107±11	112±13	116±13	119±14	121±16	122±17	123±17
迷走神经阻断组	8	135±12	122±12	125±13	127±13	128±13	130±13	132±13	133±13
自主神经阻断组	8	142±14*	129±12	135±12	136±12	137±13	139±13	139±13	140±13

* $P<0.05$ vs 对照组，△ $P<0.05$ vs 刺激前

表1-2　各组dAERP在心房快速刺激下的变化（$\bar{x} \pm s$, ms）

组别	n	刺激前	刺激时						
			1h	2h	3h	4h	5h	6h	7h
对照组	8	28±5.6	26±5.2	25±5.3	24±5.2	23±5.2	23±5.3	22±5.2	21±5.3
迷走神经阻断组	8	24±4.1	23±4.2	22±4.2	22±4.2	22±4.2	21±4.2	21±4.0	21±4.1
自主神经阻断组	8	24±4.1	23±4.1	22±4.2	22±4.2	22±4.2	22±3.9	21±4.0	21±4.1

组别	n	刺激前	刺激终止后						
			1h	2h	3h	4h	5h	6h	7h
对照组	8	28±5.6	24±5.3	27±5.5	29±5.5	32±5.6	35±5.8	38±6.7	40±7.4*
迷走神经阻断组	8	24±4.1	23±4.5	24±4.7	25±4.7	26±4.9	26±4.9	27±4.9	28±5.1
自主神经阻断组	8	24±4.1	22±4.2	24±4.3	25±4.4	26±4.6	27±4.6	27±4.7	28±5.1

* $P<0.05$ vs 快速刺激时

表1-3 HRV在对照组心房快速刺激前后的变化（$\bar{x}\pm s$, ms）

参数	刺激前			刺激终止后			
	1h	1h	2h	3h	4h	5h	6h	7h

参数	刺激前 1h	1h	2h	3h	4h	5h	6h	7h
SDNN	39±10	31±8	33±9	35±10	37±12	40±10	43±12	49±13*
SDANN	31±9	24±7	26±9	29±9	31±10	34±10	37±11*	43±11*
SDNNidx	19±7	15±6	17±7	18±7	20±8	23±8	26±10	27±9
rMSSD	13±4	10±4	12±5	12±4	15±6	17±6	19±5	25±6*
PNN$_{50\%}$	1.5±1.3	1.1±0.8	1.1±0.8	1.2±1.1	1.3±1.1	1.5±1.4	1.5±1.3	1.6±1.4

* $P<0.05$ vs 刺激终止1h后

讨 论

临床研究认为房颤是一种自身延续性疾病,尤其是阵发性房颤易转变成慢性。房颤复律后仍有部分病人易复发[9,10]。1995年 Wijffels[1]提出了房颤生成房颤的假说,并通过动物试验还提出心房电重构的概念,即心房快速刺激或短阵房颤可以使 AERP 逐渐缩短,这种 AERP 的缩短反过来可使房颤容易诱发或使原有短阵房颤转变为持续性房颤,复律为窦性心律后,缩短的 AERP 逐渐恢复延长。有学者认为在电重构中细胞内钙离子超载是一重要原因,近年来越来越多的研究发现迷走神经在电重构中有重要作用。但他们没有进一步通过阻断迷走神经来说明迷走神经高张力对快速心律失常恢复后心房电生理的直接影响。

本实验采用快速心房刺激动物模型,分析 HRV 和 AERP 来观察迷走神经张力变化与心房电重构的关系。结果发现:快速心房刺激可引起心房电重构,电重构主要表现为 AERP 缩短,而且 AERP 缩短出现较早,dAERP 无明显变化。停止刺激后 AERP 很快恢复,dAERP 明显升高。心率变异参数在刺激终止后明显升高。自主神经阻断后 AERP 明显升高。但快速刺激仍可引起电重构,dAERP 在刺激前和刺激后均无明显变化。

迷走神经对 AERP 的影响目前报道结果不一,Jalife[11]等实验刺激迷走神经或注射 Ach 可以使 AERP 明显缩短,同时房内传导发生障碍,这是引起房颤折返激动的电生理条件。Sharifov 等[12]也通过刺激迷走神经(10~50Hz)引发单个或多个房性早搏(房早)和/或房颤,随着迷走神经刺激的加强,房早和房颤的发生增加,故他们认为随着刺激迷走神经频率的升高,房早和房颤的发生率增加。迷走神经刺激引起局部异位房早在心房内分布广泛,而一个单一的房早就足以引起房颤的发生。Schauerte 等[13]通过导管介入共标测 7 处心房不同位置的 AERP,在右肺动脉的部位刺激迷走神经,7 个部位的 AERP 都明显缩短。后通过射频消融这些迷走神经均能使 AERP 明显延长。

也有学者持不同观点。Wijffels 等[14]观察了房颤电重构出现前后阿托品与普奈洛尔对 AERP 的影响,结果表明在窦性心律与房颤维持 1~3d 时,阿托品与普奈洛尔对 AERP 只产生轻微影响。房颤引起的 AERP 缩短在使用阿托品和/或普奈洛尔后仍持续存在。慢性房颤时,使用阿托品和普奈洛尔,平均房颤间期虽也轻度延长(分别为 99±5,98±10ms),但与新近发生房颤时的房颤间期(148±13ms)相比却短得多。据此作者认为,交感和迷走神经张力增加是神经递质的高敏感性,而不是房颤诱导 AERP 缩短的主要介导因素。Goette 等[15]认为自主神经对 AERP 没有明显影响。Wijffels 等[16]观察了房颤电重构出现前后阿托品与普奈洛尔对 AERP 的影响,结果表明在窦性心律与房颤维持 1~3d 时,阿托品与普奈洛尔对 AERP 只产生轻微影响。房颤引起的 AERP 缩短在使用阿托品和/或普奈洛尔后仍持续存在。

本实验中发现在基础状态下用阿托品阻断迷走神经后 AERP 改变不明显,联用阿托品和普奈洛尔阻断迷走神经和交感神经后 AERP 明显升高,与在基础状态下单用阿托品相比,AERP 无明显差异,看来交感神经与迷走神经可能具有协同缩短 AERP 的作用[17]。心率变异参数在快速刺激终止 7 h 后与刺激终止时相比明显升高,说明迷走神经张力明显升高,迷走神经张力在心房刺激前后的变化可能因为在房颤或心房快速刺激时,心脏射血分数降低,相应引起交感神经张力升高,迷走神经张力下降[18]。窦性心律恢复后,血液动力学恢复,致使迷走神经张力过度恢复[19]。

迷走神经可以使 dAERP 升高已被大多数学者认同[20,21]。Gaspo 等[22]发现快速心房起搏 42d 后,AERP 离散度升高。Liu 通过刺激麻醉犬的交感神经和双迷走神经,发现交感神经和迷走神经对 AERP 有相似的影响,但刺激迷走神经可使房颤持续时间明显延长,并且使 AERP 离散度升高;而刺激交感神经对 AERP 的离散度影响不明显。Hirose 等[23]在研究垂体的腺苷酸环化酶多肽对犬心房电生理影响时发现,迷走神经刺激可使高位右心房的 ERP 缩短,但对高位左心房、低位左心房、低位右心房无明显影响。以上资料说明,dAERP 升高是由于 AERP 恢复的空间分布不均一并与迷走神经的分布不均一有密切关系。由于迷走神经分布部位的 AERP 恢复延迟,使 AERP 离散度升高。Farch 等[24]认为心房空间分布的不同,AERP 也不同,AERP 变异性高,房颤的易损性与持续性与 AERP 或波长的关系不明显,而是与 AERP 的离散度有关,即 AERP 离散度升高是房颤发生的重要原因。

本实验中发现刺激心房前应用阿托品阻断迷走神经或联用普奈洛尔同时阻断迷走神经和交感神经后对 dAERP 却无明显影响,在快速心房刺激终止后可明显抑制 dAERP 升高,与迷走神经在快速刺激终止后的作用相比来看,迷走神经高张力才对 dAERP 有明显升高作用。正常情况下迷走神经张力对 dAERP 无明显影响,对于迷走神经张力升高多少才对 dAERP 有明显升高作用尚需进一步研究。房颤的易损性与持续性与 AERP 或波长的关系不明显,而与 AERP 的离散有关,即 AERP 离散度升高是房颤发生的重要原因[25,26]。本研究结果提示,在房颤复律后,可通过降低迷走神经张力来降低复律后的复发率。

此研究是在全麻醉下进行的,全麻醉也会对犬的自主神经产生影响,但此实验采用自身对照,并且相对药物(阿托品、普奈洛尔)对自主神经的影响很小,故全麻醉情况下对本研究结果不会产生影响,本实验中每 1 次实验时间共约 15h,刺激前后的 HRV 监测分布在上午和晚上,正常犬的 HRV 时域指标在早晚无显著差异[27]。故此结果可客观反映不同状态下对 HRV 的影响。

结 论

阻断迷走神经不能阻止电重构的发生,但迷走神经张力变化与 dAERP 有密切关系,基础状态下迷走神经张力对 dAERP 没有明显影响,而迷走神经高张力才对 dAERP 有明显升高作用,且迷走神经与交感神经对 AERP 有协同作用。

第2章 迷走神经刺激和乙酰胆碱灌注对心房肌电生理的影响

实验研究都已经证实使用 Ach 或刺激迷走神经(VS)可缩短 AERP 和心房激动的波长,增加 AERP 离散度,并能引发房颤的发生[1-3]。Ach 通过激活 G 蛋白促进心肌 K^+ 外流,心房肌折返激动是由于心房组织不应期的非均一性,这种异质性引起不应期的离散和心房折返[4,5]。Zou 等[6]在不同 Ach 浓度情况下,用二维犬心房数学模式来模拟胆碱能房颤,发现单一优势转子或多发折返旋子都能维持颤动,并与不同基质大小有关。为了进一步比较迷走神经刺激对左右心房和心耳的影响,及胺碘酮对迷走神经刺激诱发房颤的作用,我们通过 VS 和 Ach 灌注,来观察心房肌不同部位的电生理变化和诱发房颤情况,并观察应用胺碘酮后迷走神经刺激对心房肌电生理影响的变化,探讨其治疗房颤的机制。

材料与方法

1. 主要材料

   1.1 主要仪器

32 道心电生理监测仪	四川锦江产,LEAD-2000B 型
电生理刺激仪	日本产,SEN-7103 型,
电子秤	瑞典,AE200S
程序快速刺激仪	苏州产,DF-5A 型
电极操纵器	日本产,UNM-1 型

1.2 主要试剂

乙酰胆碱针剂	上海三爱思试剂有限公司
胺碘酮针剂	杭州赛诺菲民生公司
甲醛	上海三爱思试剂有限公司
戊巴比妥钠	上海三爱思试剂有限公司

2. 实验对象

2004年5月—2004年7月由武汉大学人民医院动物房提供成年杂种犬10只，雌雄不拘，体重17～22kg。

3. 实验方法

3.1 动物准备

戊巴比妥钠30 mg/kg腹腔麻醉（根据动物反应每30～60 min静脉追加戊巴比妥钠50 mg），气管插管，人工通气，麻醉后左右侧颈部备皮（10 cm×10 cm），胸壁备皮（20 cm×10 cm）。固定手术床，常规消毒铺巾。经胸骨行正中开胸术，切开心包，暴露心脏，缝制心包吊床。右侧股静脉以0.9%生理盐水维持静脉通路，采用体表Ⅱ、aVF、aVR导联监测心电图。

3.2 电极放置与电生理检查

取6根包被有聚四氟乙烯的银针，其中3根为一组，由一橡胶条制成梳状电极，间距约1cm左右，制备的电极由电极操纵器固定在心房肌外膜，包括右心耳（RAA）、高位右心房（HRA）、低位右心房（LRA）、左心耳（LAA）、高位左心房（HLA）、低位左心房（LLA），参比电极固定于犬胸壁皮下。引出的单相动作电位（MAP）经直流电前置放大器放大后输入32道心电生理监测仪，共计录6个不同部位的MAP。

3.3 刺激神经与分组

10只犬采用自身对照。其中每只犬在开胸的同时，分离左右颈部迷走神经干，切断双侧迷走神经（0.2mg/kg 普奈洛尔静注阻断交感神经），用刺激电极插入双侧迷走神经末端。先记录心房6个不同部位的 MAP，然后用电生理刺激仪，以刺激频率 20Hz 和 0.2ms 的刺激波宽，10V 的电压刺激迷走神经干远端，同时观察心率的变化和记录心房 6 个不同部位的 MAP；停止 VS_1，待心房 MAP 和心率完全恢复后，用电生理刺激仪，以刺激频率 20Hz 和 0.2ms 的刺激波宽，30V 的电压刺激迷走神经干远端，同时观察心率的变化和记录心房 6 个不同部位的 MAP；停止 VS_2，待心房 MAP 和心率完全恢复后，钳夹阻断升主动脉 2~3s，同时于主动脉根部注入 Ach 20~60μmol/L，使 Ach 灌注到冠状动脉，注入的剂量以引起心率的变化与 VS_1 基本相同为宜，同时记录心房 6 个不同部位的 MAP；待心房 MAP 和心率完全恢复后，静脉注入胺碘酮 1mg/kg，5min 后再次 VS_1。由于在体心率不恒定，实验中心动周期实测值按均数±标准差处理，犬在双侧迷走神经切断后心动周期为 300±32ms，按 300ms 处理；VS_1 和 Ach 灌注后心动周期分别为 810±40ms，800±36ms，均认为心率减慢程度相同。其中在 VS_1 前、VS_1 时、VS_2 时、VS_1+胺碘酮时灌注 Ach 时，在右心耳给一电刺激，观察诱发房颤的情况。把每只犬在基础状态下的 MAP 记录作为对照组；每只犬在 VS_1 状态下完成的 MAP 记录作为 VS_1 组；每只犬在 VS_2 状态下完成的 MAP 记录作为 VS_2 组；每只犬在灌注 Ach 状态下完成的 MAP 记录作为 Ach 灌注组；每只犬在 VS_1+胺碘酮状态下完成的 MAP 记录作为 VS_1+胺碘酮组。五组均于记录 MAP 图形时，同步记录心电图。

3.4 观察和测量指标

① 观察各组诱发房早和房颤的情况。

② 动作电位时程（APD）参数：APD_{50} 为 MAP 从 0 期至复极到 50% 的时程；APD_{90} 为 MAP 从 0 期至复极到 90% 的时程。

③ APD 离散度（dAPD）：心房 6 个部位最大 APD 值与最小 APD 值的差值。

3.5 统计学处理

实验数据以均数±标准差表示，采用 t 检验和方差分析统计结果，以 $P<0.05$ 为差异有显著性。

结　果

1. 各组中诱发房早、房颤的情况

对照组有 2 例诱发房早，无一例诱发出房颤；VS_1 组 10 只犬 7 例诱发房颤，诱发率为 70%；VS_2 组 10 只犬 8 例诱发房颤，诱发率为 80%；Ach 灌注组 10 只犬 6 例诱发房颤，诱发率为 60%；VS_1 +胺碘酮组 10 只犬诱发 2 例房颤，诱发率为 20%。

2. 各组心外膜 MAP 时程长短的变化

对照组，犬心房肌外膜的 MAP 1 期复极迅速，呈尖峰状，没有明显的平台期，心房肌不同部位在 APD_{90} 有离散的趋势，RAA 的 APD_{90} 为 $136\pm7ms$，LLA 的 APD_{90} 为 $131\pm6ms$；

VS_1 组，心房 6 个部位 APD_{50} 和 APD_{90} 与对照组相比均明显缩短，MAP 呈明显的倒三角形，没有平台期。其中 RAA 缩短最明显，APD_{50} 从 $72\pm5ms$ 到 $19\pm4ms$，APD_{90} 从 $136\pm7ms$ 到 $43\pm5ms$（$P<0.001$）；

VS_2 组，心房 6 个部位 APD_{50} 和 APD_{90} 与对照组相比也均明显缩短，其中 RAA 的 APD_{50} 从 $72\pm5ms$ 到 $17\pm4ms$，APD_{90} 从 $136\pm7ms$ 到 $38\pm5ms$（$P<0.001$）

Ach 灌注组，心房 6 个部位 APD_{50} 和 APD_{90} 与对照组相比也明显缩短，MAP 形状与 VS 组基本相同，但与 VS_1 组相比，LLA 的 APD_{90} 缩短更明显（$53\pm6ms$ 比 $62\pm8ms$，$P<0.01$）；

VS_1 +胺碘酮组，心房 6 个部位 APD_{50} 和 APD_{90} 与对照组相比也明显缩短，但与 VS 相比，明显延长（图 2-1、图 2-2、图 2-4、表 2-1、表 2-2）。

3. 各组心外膜 dAPD 的变化

五组 dAPD 在 APD_{50} 和 APD_{90} 的比较，APD_{50} 时，VS_1 与对照组相比，dAPD 明显升高（$11\pm5ms$ 比 $5\pm3ms$，$P<0.01$），VS_2、Ach

灌注组和 VS_1 + 胺碘酮组与对照组相比没有差别；APD_{90} 时，VS_1 组和 Ach 灌注组的 dAPD 均比对照组明显升高（$19 \pm 7ms$，$15 \pm 7ms$ 比 $7 \pm 5ms$，$P < 0.01$）；但 VS_2 组和 VS_1 + 胺碘酮组与对照组相比没有差别（图 2-3、表 2-3）。

表 2-1

部位	n	对照组	VS_1 组	VS_2 组	Ach 灌注组	VS_1 + 胺碘酮组
RAA	10	72 ± 6	$19 \pm 4^*$	$17 \pm 4^*$	$20 \pm 4^*$	$60 \pm 4^\Delta$
HRA	10	68 ± 5	$22 \pm 4^*$	$20 \pm 4^*$	$21 \pm 4^*$	$58 \pm 4^\Delta$
LRA	10	67 ± 4	$29 \pm 5^*$	$23 \pm 5^*$	$24 \pm 5^*$	$55 \pm 5^\Delta$
LAA	10	69 ± 5	$20 \pm 4^*$	$19 \pm 4^*$	$19 \pm 3^*$	$59 \pm 5^\Delta$
HLA	10	68 ± 4	$23 \pm 4^*$	$22 \pm 4^*$	$22 \pm 4^*$	$57 \pm 4^\Delta$
LLA	10	67 ± 5	$30 \pm 6^*$	$24 \pm 6^*$	$25 \pm 5^*$	$54 \pm 4^\Delta$

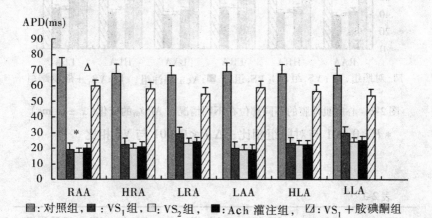

■：对照组，■：VS_1 组，□：VS_2 组，■：Ach 灌注组，▨：VS_1 + 胺碘酮组

图 2-1 心房肌外膜的不同部位在不同情况下 APD_{50} 的变化（$\bar{x} \pm s$, ms）
＊$P < 0.001$ vs 对照组；Δ $P < 0.001$ vs VS 组。

表 2-2

部位	n	对照组	VS_1组	VS_2组	Ach 灌注组	VS_1 + 胺碘酮组
RAA	10	136 ± 7	43 ± 5*	38 ± 4*	39 ± 4*	120 ± 5△
HRA	10	134 ± 8	48 ± 6*	42 ± 5*	42 ± 5*	122 ± 6△
LRA	10	132 ± 6	61 ± 7*	47 ± 6*	54 ± 6*	116 ± 6△
LAA	10	133 ± 7	44 ± 5*	40 ± 4*	40 ± 5*	122 ± 7△
HLA	10	132 ± 6	51 ± 6*	45 ± 5*	42 ± 5*	118 ± 6△
LLA	10	129 ± 6	62 ± 8*	46 ± 6*	53 ± 6*	115 ± 5△

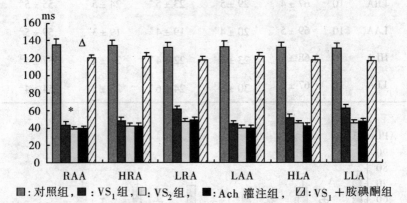

■: 对照组, ■: VS_1组, □: VS_2组, ■: Ach 灌注组, ▨: VS_1 + 胺碘酮组

图 2-2　心房肌外膜的不同部位在不同情况下 APD_{90} 的变化($\bar{x} \pm s$, ms)

*$P < 0.001$ 与对照组相比；△$P < 0.001$ 与 VS 相比

表 2-3

部位	对照组	VS_1组	VS_2组	Ach 灌注组	VS_1 + 胺碘酮组
APD_{50}	5 ± 3	11 ± 5*	7 ± 5	6 ± 5	6 ± 5
APD_{90}	7 ± 5	19 ± 7*△	9 ± 6	15 ± 7*	7 ± 6

第2章 迷走神经刺激和乙酰胆碱灌注对心房肌电生理的影响

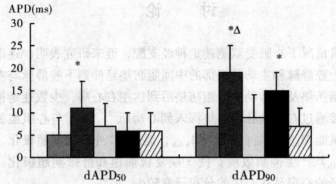

图2-3 心房肌外膜在不同情况下dAPD的变化（$\bar{x} \pm s$, ms）
*$P<0.01$ vs 对照组，$^\triangle P<0.01$ vs VS_2组。

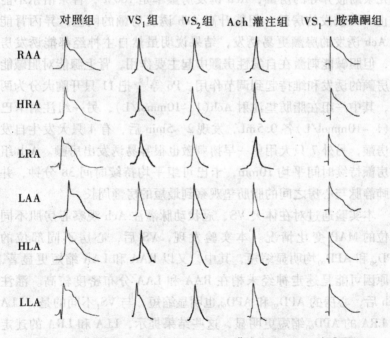

图2-4 对照组、VS_1组、VS_2组、Ach灌注组和VS_1+胺碘酮组不同部位的MAP比较

讨 论

正常情况下心脏受双侧迷走神经支配，近来研究表明，迷走神经通过上腔静脉和主动脉根部的中间脂肪垫延伸到下腔静脉与左房之间的脂肪垫及右肺动脉的脂肪垫后到达左右心房，少数迷走神经纤维直接通过右肺动脉脂肪垫深入到心房肌[7]，Ach 与心肌细胞膜上的胆碱能 M_2 受体结合，激活 I_{KAch}，促进 K^+ 外流使膜超极化。对 I_K，I_f，I_{Ca} 均产生抑制效应，使 3 期复极加速和舒张期超极化。但迷走神经的心房丛在心房的分布研究较少。

Sharifov 等[8]在 20 只犬通过窦房结动脉灌注儿茶酚胺类或 Ach 及儿茶酚胺类和 Ach 混合物，比较诱发房颤的情况，发现异丙肾和肾上腺素诱发房颤率分别为 21% 和 17%，应用阿托品后可以阻止儿茶酚胺介导的房颤；Ach 诱发房颤率是 100%，普奈洛尔不能阻止 Ach 诱发的房颤，但能升高 Ach 诱发房颤的阈值，异丙肾能使 Ach 诱发的房颤更易诱发，结果说明虽然自主神经都能诱发房颤，但胆碱能刺激在自发性房颤中起主要作用，肾上腺能对胆碱能性房颤的诱发和维持起到调节作用。Po 等[9]把 11 只开胸犬分为两组，其中一组在脂肪垫注射 Ach(1~10mmol/L)，另一组注射卡巴可(1~10mmol/L)各 0.5mL，发现 2~5min 后，有 4 只犬发生自发性房颤，另外 7 只犬用单一早搏刺激也很容易诱发出房颤。Ach 组的房颤持续时间平均 10min，卡巴可组平均持续时间 38 分钟，并在肺静脉与心房之间的脂肪垫观察到最短的房颤周长。

本实验通过对在体犬 VS、冠状动脉灌注 Ach 观察心房肌不同部位的 MAP 变化情况。本实验发现，VS 后，心房不同部位的 APD_{50} 和 APD_{90} 均明显缩短，其中，又以 RAA 和 LAA 缩短更显著，其原因可能是迷走神经末梢在 RAA 和 LAA 分布密度较高。灌注 Ach 后，心房的 APD_{50} 和 APD_{90} 也明显缩短，与 VS_1 不同的是，LLA 和 LRA 的 APD_{90} 缩短更明显，这些结果提示，LLA 和 LRA 的迷走神经末梢分布可能与 M 受体分布不成比例。心房肌细胞的复极过程有多种离子参与，其中 2 期主要是 I_{Ca} 内流和 I_K 外流，3 期主要是

I_{KAch}和I_{K1}外流，本实验发现 VS 和 Ach 灌注后心房肌 APD_{50} 均明显缩短，说明迷走神经兴奋和 Ach 灌注对 I_{Ca} 的抑制作用也有关。

近来研究证明通过对副交感神经末梢在心房不同部位的刺激释放 Ach 所引起的 AERP 离散足以导致折返，并且静注或灌注 Ach 或卡巴可或腺苷都能引发房速的发生[10]。但如果心房内缺少 Ach 则不能发生房颤[11]，迷走神经兴奋可能会诱发折返机制的房颤。但 Wang 等[12]发现在猫心房肌 Ach 的减少能改变膜电位、升高 I_{CaL} 的钙离子流，并引起肌质网细胞内钙离子超载，导致心房肌细胞的延迟后除极，认为这种机制可能是由于迷走神经活动的消失引起房性早期除极，然而这种机制并不能解释为什么房性早期除极发生在胆碱能刺激存在时。在我们的研究过程中，大多数房颤发生在 Ach 灌注或 VS 时，而不是在恢复时。在另一个研究中，Fedorov 和他的同事证实维拉帕米静脉注射后对 Ach 灌注引起的房颤也无影响，表明这种自发性触发与细胞内 Ca^{2+} 超载无关。

目前研究认为刺激迷走神经诱发房颤的原因是由于 APD 离散，导致折返的发生[13-16]，通过降低波长及增加多个折返环路发生的几率，从而使房颤的维持更稳定[17]。Hirose 等[18]在 12 例孤立犬右心房用高分析光标技术监测 APD，直接比较灌注 Ach 和刺激迷走神经对房速诱发的影响，发现 Ach 组的 APD 明显比迷走神经刺激组和对照组缩短，应用 Ach 后单一提前刺激很易引发房速，同样在迷走神经刺激组也有同样发现。与 Ach 组相比，迷走神经刺激组升高极化恢复的离散，与传导阻滞和不完全折返有关，但是在相同的心房组织结构和起搏部位直接注射 Ach 却很少发现有传导阻滞发生，这可能与迷走神经在心房的分布不均有关。本实验发现，VS_1 明显升高心房肌细胞 APD_{50} 和 APD_{90} 的离散，但在 VS_2 组 APD 离散与对照组相比却没有明显差异，而 VS_1 组和 VS_2 组都能明显诱发房颤，结果提示，APD 缩短是 VS 诱发房颤的基础，即使 APD 离散没有升高，单独 APD 缩短就可足以诱发房颤。乙酰胆碱灌注虽然缩短 APD，与对照组相比，$dAPD_{90}$ 也明显升高，可能的原因是虽然迷走神经在心房的分布不均一，并且 M_2 受体和 I_{KAch} 通道在心房的分布可能也不一致。

胺碘酮是治疗房颤较好的药物，研究认为胺碘酮对CCh、腺苷和GTP-γ-S引起I_{KAch}的阻断作用基本相似，说明胺碘酮主要作用于K_{Ach}通道或GTP结合蛋白，而不是M_2受体[19,20]，但胺碘酮不是一个选择性的通道阻断剂，它可以抑制I_{KAch}和几个内向电流($I_{Ca,L}$)和外向电流(I_{Kr}，I_{Ks}，I_{Ki})。本实验发现VS和Ach灌注均易诱发房颤，而VS_1+胺碘酮后房颤诱发率明显降低，但与对照组相比仍有2例诱发房颤，说明胺碘酮虽然能降低迷走神经刺激诱发房颤率，但不能完全阻断迷走神经刺激诱发房颤的作用。胺碘酮能明显降低VS对心房肌APD的影响，并能降低APD的离散，胺碘酮的这种作用可能是其降低迷走神经刺激诱发房颤率的机制。

结 论

VS和Ach灌注都易诱发房颤的发生，并且对心耳APD的影响较大；VS诱发房颤的基础主要是APD缩短，VS引起APD离散与VS的强度有关；胺碘酮能有效地降低迷走神经刺激诱发房颤。

第3章 胆碱能 M_2 受体和乙酰胆碱敏感钾通道在心房肌及其相邻大静脉的分布研究

迷走神经对心房肌的影响是通过其末梢释放的递质 Ach 作用于胆碱能 M_2 受体，与 G 蛋白结合后激活 K_{Ach} 通道，促进 K^+ 外流，使膜超极化，使3期复极加速和舒张期超极化，增大舒张期电位与阈电位距离。心房内神经支配的不均一可能是迷走神经刺激导致房颤的重要原因，有学者研究发现 Kir3.4 和 Kir3.1mRNAs 在左房比右房丰富，并认为这种差异是导致迷走神经刺激引起心房内折返的机制。目前研究发现诱发房颤的大多数异位兴奋灶在肺静脉内，也可存在上腔静脉、界嵴和左房后游离壁等[1~8]，近来报道消融肺静脉的异位兴奋灶和迷走神经比单独消融异位兴奋灶房颤的复发率明显降低[4]。为了进一步探讨 M_2 受体和 K_{Ach} 通道在心房的分布及其与异位兴奋灶的关系，我们通过 Western-blot 检测 M_2 受体蛋白，用膜片钳技术来观察 IK_{Ach} 在心房及其相邻大静脉的分布情况，并研究胺碘酮对 IK_{Ach} 的影响。

材料与方法

1. 主要材料

1.1 主要仪器

32 道心电生理监测仪　　　四川锦江产，LEAD-2000B 型
电生理刺激仪　　　　　　日本产，SEN-7103 型，

磁力恒温搅拌器	774 型，江苏医疗器械厂
倒置显微镜	IMT-2，Olympus，Japan
三维式液压微操纵器	MO-203，NARISHIGE
微电极拉制器	PP-83，NARISHIGE
微电极抛光器	MF-9，NARISHIGE
电热恒温水浴箱	上海医疗器械厂
电子秤	瑞典，AE200S
垂直电泳槽	BIO-RAD 公司；
转移电泳仪	北京六一仪器厂
稳压稳流电泳仪	DYY-6B 型
电源控制器	Biometra 公司。
膜片钳系统	
电极支持系统	日本 Nihon 公司
膜片钳负反馈放大器	HEKA EPC9　德国 HEKA 公司
数/膜转换器	Digidat1200　日本 Nihon 公司
P400 型计算机	美国 Compaq 公司
Pulse + Pulsefit 软件	德国 HEKA 公司
（version8.31）	

1.2 主要试剂

氯化钠
氯化钾
氯化镁
氯化钙
磷酸二氢钠
HEPES
葡萄糖　　　　均为国产分析纯，购自
甘露醇　　　　上海化学试剂采购供应站
EGTA
磷酸二氢钾
小牛血清白蛋白
氢氧化钾
氢氧化钠
氯化镉

肝素钠	
胶原酶Ⅱ	均为国产分析纯，购自
乙酰胆碱	上海化学试剂采购供应站
胆碱	

M_2一抗	Santa Cruz 公司;
辣根酶标记山羊抗兔的二抗	Pirece 公司;
Bradford 比色试剂盒	BioRad 公司;
NC 膜	pharmacia 公司;

potassium glutamate	
β-hydroxybutyric acid	
taurine	
potassium aspartate	
Mg-ATP	
GTP	购自 Sigma 公司
phosphocreatine	
Glyburide	
chromanol 293B	
pirenzepine	
tropicamide	
4-DAMP	

E-4031　　　购自 Alexis 公司

2. 实验对象

2004 年 11 月—2005 年 9 月由武汉大学人民医院动物房提供成年杂种犬 30 只，雌雄不拘，体重 15~20kg。

3. 实验方法

3.1 实验分组

戊巴比妥钠 30 mg/kg 腹腔麻醉，气管插管，人工通气，麻醉后左右侧颈部备皮(10 cm×10 cm)。固定手术床，常规消毒铺巾。右侧股静脉以 0.9% 生理盐水维持静脉通路，采用体表Ⅱ、aVF、aVR 导联监测心电图。分离左右颈部迷走神经干，切断双侧迷走神经，用刺激电极插入双侧迷走神经末端。用电生理刺激仪，以刺激频率 20Hz 和 0.2ms 的刺激波宽，10～30V 的电压刺激迷走神经干远端，通过心电图观察诱发房颤情况，其中诱发房颤的犬作为房颤组，未能诱发房颤的犬作为对照组。

3.2 Western-blot 检测
3.2.1 标本收集
迷走神经刺激后，开胸取出心脏，分别取左右心耳、左右心房、肺静脉和腔静脉。

3.2.2 SDS-PAGE 凝胶的灌制
a) 无水乙醇清洗并烘干玻璃板后，按仪器说明书安装；
b) 配制 10% 分离胶溶液 5mL，迅速灌注于两玻璃板间，留出积层胶所需空间(Teflon 梳子的齿长再加 2cm)，用胶头吸管小心于其上覆盖一层无水乙醇，室温放置约 30min；
c) 分离胶聚合完全后，倾出覆盖层液体，用去离子水洗涤凝胶顶部以除去未聚合的丙稀酰胺，用滤纸条吸尽残液；
d) 配制积层胶 3mL，在分离胶上直接灌注积层胶，立即将 Teflon 梳子插入玻璃板间积层胶中，室温放置 30min；
e) 积层胶聚合完全凝固后，小心拔除梳子，用去离子水洗涤上样孔，以除去未聚合的聚丙烯酰胺。

3.2.3 上样、电泳
a) 每样本蛋白取 50μg，加入样本体积 1/2 的 3×SDS-PAGE 上样缓冲液，然后用 1×SDS-PAGE 上样缓冲液补足至总体积 25μL 混匀后煮沸 5min，以微量上样器每孔上样 20μL。
b) 接通电源(正极接下槽)，所加电压为 8V/cm。当溴酚蓝染料前沿进入分离胶后，电压提高至 15V/cm，溴酚蓝染料达到分离胶底部时关闭电源中断电泳。
c) 取出玻璃板，切除积层胶，小心取下分离胶并做好方向标记。

3.2.4 蛋白质电转移和膜封闭

a) 剪切一张 NC 膜和两张 Wortman 滤纸，其大小与分离胶相当，并做好方向标记；

b) 将 NC 膜置入电转缓冲液中浸泡 5min，滤纸在使用前临时置入电转缓冲液中浸湿；

c) 依次将滤纸-凝胶-NC 膜-滤纸平铺于支撑垫上，逐层叠放，并用玻璃棒赶出其间气泡，闭合支架，将其置入充满电转缓冲液转膜电泳槽中，接通电源，25V 转印 2h；转印结束后，用考马斯亮蓝染液染胶，检查蛋白质转移是否完全；

d) 转印完成后将 NC 膜取出用铅笔标记或剪角以标记方向，用 15mLTBS 缓冲液浸洗 NC 膜 5min，将 NC 膜置含 5% 脱脂奶粉的膜封闭液中封闭 90min（室温，摇床上平缓摇动）。

3.2.5 抗原抗体反应

a) 用 TBST 漂洗 NC 膜 4 次，每次在室温下振荡 15min；

b) 加入一抗浓度（1:200）（即 30μL M_2 +6mL TBST）温育 2h；

c) 再用 TBST 液漂洗 4 次，每次 15min；

d) 再加辣根酶标记山羊抗兔的二抗（1:5000）（20mLTBST+4μL 二抗）温育 1h。再漂洗，摇匀 4 次，每次 15min；

e) 显色，DAB 试剂盒。

3.2.6 摄像

凝胶共聚成分系统进行分析（VL.France，Vilber 公司）

试剂配制：

1. 分离胶缓冲液（pH=8.8）：1.5mol/L Tris Base，0.4% SDS，去离子水；

2. 积层胶缓冲液（pH=6.8）：0.5mol/L Tris Base，0.4% SDS，去离子水；

3. 30% 丙稀酰胺（PPA）溶液（100mL）：29.2200g 丙稀酰胺+0.7792g 甲叉双丙稀酰胺加水至 100mL，加热至 37℃，溶解后室温避光保存；

4. 10% 过硫酸铵（AMPS）溶液（10mL）：过硫酸铵 1g 加水至

10mL溶解，4℃储存，一周内用；

5. 10×TBS缓冲液（100mL，pH = 7.6）：2.42g Tris Base + 8.18g NaCl加水至100mL；

6. TBS/T缓冲液：1×TBS缓冲液加入0.1%Tween20；

7. 膜封闭液（50mL）：0.25mL Tween20 + 2.5g脱脂奶粉完全溶于50mL 1×TBS溶液。

3.3 K_{Ach}电流记录

3.3.1 单个心肌细胞的分离

用500IU/kg肝素钠静脉注射抗凝后迅速开胸取出心脏，在100%氧饱和的0℃生理盐水中挤压排除腔内残血。小心分离，操作过程保持在上述液体中。在37℃100%氧饱和恒温无钙台氏液中将右心耳组织剪碎成1mm³大小组织块，冲洗3次，每次5~6min。弃上清液后将组织块置于37℃恒温100%氧饱和含150~300IU/mL胶原酶Ⅱ、0.1%小牛血清白蛋白（BSA）的低钙台氏液（钙浓度为125μmol/L）中孵育，以磁力搅拌，30~45min后弃除含酶液并更换新的消化液，尔后每隔5~10min取样观察，在单个心肌细胞的数量与质量达到最佳时，将含0.1%BSA的低钙台氏液稀释4倍后，去除大的组织块获得单个心肌细胞悬液并逐渐复钙，于室温下保留备用。剩余组织块采用同样浓度的新鲜酶液消化，同法收集并保存细胞。左心耳、左右心房、肺静脉和上腔静脉的单个细胞分离同上[9]。

3.3.2 全细胞膜片钳记录

按Hamill等方法进行全细胞膜片钳记录实验。吸数滴上述细胞悬液加入细胞池中，置于倒置显微镜工作台上，待细胞沉底附壁后，细胞外液以BPS-4灌流装置灌流，流速1~1.5mL/min，温度保持22~26℃。利用三维式液压微操纵器移动电极选择边缘整齐、表面无颗粒、横纹清晰、无收缩的细胞，用负压使电极尖端与细胞膜之间形成1GΩ以上的高阻抗封接，补偿快电容并吸破细胞膜形成全细胞记录模式，调节慢电容补偿和串联补偿以减少瞬时充放电电流和钳位误差。脉冲信号由Pulse + Pulsefit软件控制，经EPC-9放大器放大后通过Ag-AgCl电极丝和填充电极内液的玻璃微电极导入细胞,产生的电流信号经 EPC-9 转换,存储于计算机硬盘中,供测量及分析用。

玻璃毛坯(上海神经研究所)经微电极拉制器两步法拉制成尖端为 1~1.5μm 的微电极,以抛光器抛光,充灌电极内液,入水后阻抗 2.5~6.0MΩ。

3.3.3 溶液与试剂配制

台氏液成分(mmol/L):NaCl 136;KCl 5.4;$MgCl_2$ 1.0;$CaCl_2$ 1.0;NaH_2PO_4 0.33;HEPES 5;Glucose 10;pH 值用 NaOH 调至 7.4;

无钙台氏液即上述溶液中不含 $CaCl_2$。

KB 液成分(mmol/L):KCl 20;KH_2PO_4 10;Glucose 25;potassium glutamate 70;β-hydroxybutyric acid 10;taurine 20;EGTA 10;白蛋白 0.1%;甘露醇 40;pH 值用 KOH 调至 7.4。

记录 K_{Ach} 电流的电极内液成分(mmol/L):potassium aspartate 110;KCl 20;$MgCl_2$ 1;Mg-ATP 5;GTP 0.1;EGTA 10;phosphocreatine 5;HEPES 10;pH 值用 KOH 调至 7.3。

记录 K_{Ach} 电流的细胞外液成分(mmol/L):NaCl 136;KCl 5.4;$MgCl_2$ 1.0;$CaCl_2$ 1.0;HEPES 10;Glucose 10;pH 值用 NaOH 调至 7.4。

记录 K_{Ach} 电流时在电极外液加入 CdCl(200μmol/L)阻断钙电流和钙激活的氯电流;用 Glyburide(10μmol/L)和电极内液的 Mg-ATP(5mmol/L)阻断 ATP 敏感钾通道;chromanol 293B(20μmol/L)和 E-4031(5μmol/L)分别阻断 IKs 和 IKr 通道;pirenzepine,4-DAMP 和 tropicamide 分别阻断 M_1,M_3 和 M_4 受体;I_{KAch} 由 Ach(1μmol/L)激活;预钳制电压在 -50mV 使钠电流失活[10]。

4. 统计学处理

实验数据以均数 ± 标准差表示,数据用 SPSS 软件分析,两组比较采用 t 检验,多组间用方差分析统计结果,离子流的大小以钳制电压下电流与细胞膜电容的比值(pA/pF)表示,以 $P < 0.05$ 为差异有显著性。

结 果

1. Western-blot 分析结果

房颤组：M_2受体蛋白在左心耳、右心耳、左心房的分布明显高于右心房、肺静脉和上腔静脉（光密度相对值：0.66 ± 0.08，0.67 ± 0.08 and 0.51 ± 0.06 vs 0.35 ± 0.04，0.33 ± 0.04 and 0.32 ± 0.03 $P < 0.05$），左右心耳和左心房分别比右心房的 M_2 受体分布高 88%、92% 和 45%。而且左右心耳的分布也比左心房高（0.66 ± 0.08，0.67 ± 0.08 vs 0.51 ± 0.06 $P < 0.05$）（图 3-1）。

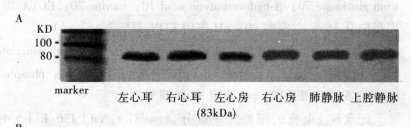

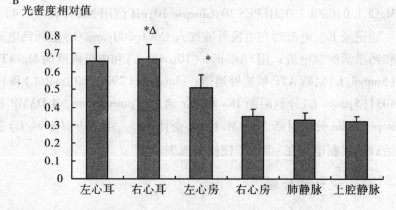

图 3-1 房颤组：M_2受体在左心耳、右心耳、左心房、右心房、肺静脉和上腔静脉的表达

* $P < 0.05$ 与右心房、肺静脉和上腔静脉相比；$^\Delta P < 0.05$ 左心房相比

对照组:M_2受体蛋白在左心耳、右心耳、左心房的分布也明显高于右心房、肺静脉和上腔静脉(光密度相对值:0.52 ± 0.06,0.53 ± 0.06 and 0.50 ± 0.05 vs 0.34 ± 0.04,0.31 ± 0.03 and 0.32 ± 0.03,$P < 0.05$),但左右心耳的分布与左心房没有明显差异(0.52 ± 0.06,0.53 ± 0.06 vs 0.50 ± 0.05 $P > 0.05$)(图3-2)。

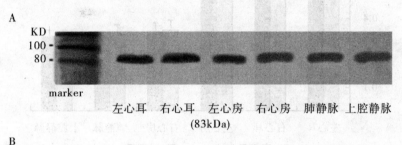

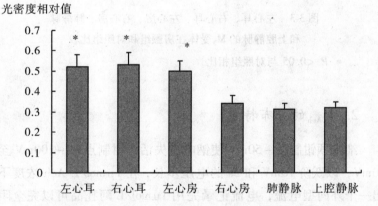

图3-2 对照组:M_2受体在左心耳、右心耳、左心房、右心房、肺静脉和上腔静脉的表达

* $P < 0.05$ 与右心房、肺静脉和上腔静脉相比。

房颤组与对照组相比,左心耳和右心耳的M_2受体分布在房颤组也比对照组高(0.66 ± 0.08 vs 0.52 ± 0.06;0.67 ± 0.08 vs 0.53 ± 0.06,$P < 0.05$)(图3-3)。

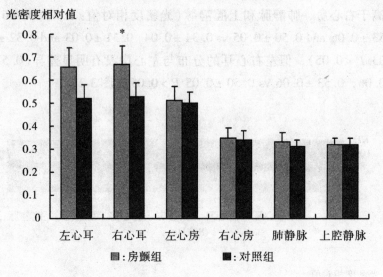

图 3-3 左心耳、右心耳、左心房、右心房、肺静脉
和上腔静脉的 M_2 受体在房颤组和对照组比较
* $P < 0.05$ 与对照组相比

2. I_{KAch} 的分布特点

细胞预钳制在 $-50mV$ 使钠电流失活,钳制点在 $-100mV$ 至 $+50mV$,以跃阶 $10mV$ 和 $2s$ 的电压步长,在 $1\mu mol/L$ Ach 浓度下引出一个外向型电流,电流记录完用 $1\mu mol/L$ 阿托品可以完全阻断此电流,证明此电流是 I_{KAch}。记录心耳、心房、肺静脉和上腔静脉的 I_{KAch} 幅值强度以 $2s$ 电压步长末时计算。这些部位的 I_{KAch} 都表现出强的内向整流性,在超极化有逐渐升高的内向电流,而在去极化表现快速衰减的外向电流。

房颤组:在 $-100mV$,左右心耳的 I_{KAch} 分别为 20.36 ± 0.91 (pA/pF, $n=6$) 和 21.23 ± 0.95 (pA/pF, $n=6$);左右心房的 I_{KAch} 分别为 14.17 ± 0.65 (pA/pF, $n=5$) 和 10.34 ± 0.62 (pA/pF, $n=6$);肺静脉和上腔静脉的 I_{KAch} 分别为 8.24 ± 0.45 (pA/pF, $n=6$) 和

7.65±0.42（pA/pF，$n=7$）。左右心耳和左心房的 I_{KAch} 强度明显比右心房、肺静脉和上腔静脉大，而且左右心耳的电流密度也比左心房大（20.36±0.91，21.23±0.95 vs 14.17±0.65，$P<0.05$）（图3-4、图3-5）。

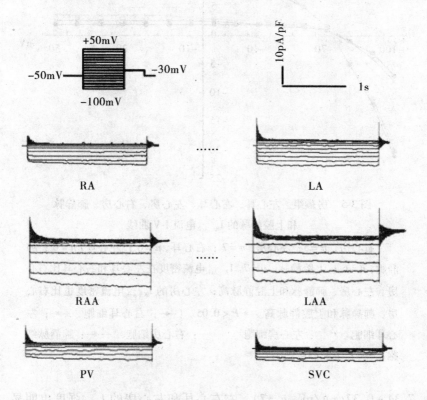

图3-4 房颤组：左心耳、右心耳、左心房、右心房、
肺静脉和上腔静脉的 $I_{K,Ach}$ 密度比较
（虚线表示零电位水平）

对照组：在 -100mV，左右心耳的 I_{KAch} 分别为 16.27±0.87（pA/pF，$n=6$）和 16.75±0.82（pA/pF，$n=6$）；左右心房的 I_{KAch} 分别为 14.78±0.63（pA/pF，$n=5$）和 10.65±0.48（pA/pF，$n=6$）；肺静脉和上腔静脉的 I_{KAch} 分别为 8.35±0.41（pA/pF，$n=6$）和

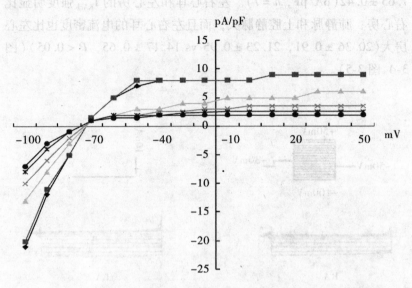

图 3-5 房颤组：左心耳、右心耳、左心房、右心房、肺静脉和上腔静脉的 $I_{K,Ach}$ 电流 I-V 曲线

右心房，$n=5$；左心房，$n=7$；右心耳，$n=6$；左心耳，$n=6$；肺静脉，$n=6$；上腔静脉，$n=7$。$I_{K,Ach}$ 电流密度在左心耳和右心耳比右心房、左心房、肺静脉和上腔静脉高；左心房的 $I_{K,Ach}$ 电流密度也比右心房、肺静脉和上腔静脉高。 $*P<0.05$。（—●—：右心耳细胞 —■—：左心耳细胞 —▲—：左心房细胞 —✳—：右心房细胞 —✕—：肺静脉细胞 —◆—：上腔静脉细胞）

7.34 ± 0.37（pA/pF，$n=7$）。左右心耳和左心房的 I_{KAch} 强度也明显比右心房、肺静脉和上腔静脉大，但左右心耳和左心房的电流密度没有明显差异（16.27 ± 0.87，16.75 ± 0.82 vs 14.78 ± 0.63，$P<0.05$）（图3-6）。

房颤组应用胺碘酮后：在 -100mV，左右心耳的 I_{KAch} 分别为 10.31 ± 0.64（pA/pF，$n=6$）和 9.84 ± 0.68（pA/pF，$n=6$）；左右心房的 I_{KAch} 分别为 6.86 ± 0.51（pA/pF，$n=5$）和 6.67 ± 0.59（pA/pF，$n=6$）；肺静脉和上腔静脉的 I_{KAch} 分别为 5.57 ± 0.39（pA/pF，

第3章 胆碱能 M_2 受体和乙酰胆碱敏感钾通道在心房肌及其相邻大静脉的分布研究

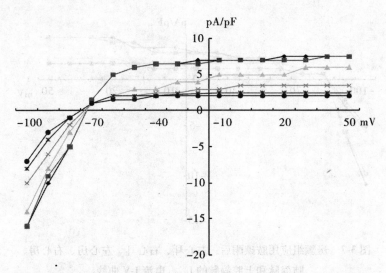

图 3-6 对照组：左心耳、右心耳、左心房、右心房、肺静脉和上腔静脉的 $I_{K,Ach}$ 电流 I-V 曲线

右心房，$n=6$；左心房，$n=6$；右心耳，$n=7$；左心耳，$n=5$；肺静脉，$n=7$；上腔静脉，$n=5$。$I_{K,Ach}$ 电流密度在左心耳、右心耳和左心房比右心房、肺静脉和上腔静脉高；左心房的 $I_{K,Ach}$ 电流密度也比右心房、肺静脉和上腔静脉高。* $P<0.05$。(●：右心耳细胞 ■：左心耳细胞 ▲：左心房细胞 ✕：右心房细胞 ✱：肺静脉细胞 ●：上腔静脉细胞)

$n=6$) 和 5.12 ± 0.34 (pA/pF, $n=7$)。胺碘酮能明显降低 I_{KAch}，左右心耳的 I_{KAch} 强度仍比左右心房、肺静脉和上腔静脉大，但左右心房的电流密度没有明显差异(6.86 ± 0.51 vs 6.67 ± 0.59，$P<0.05$)(图 3-7)。

房颤组与对照组相比，左心耳和右心耳的 I_{KAch} 密度在房颤组也比对照组高(20.36 ± 0.91 vs 16.27 ± 0.87；21.23 ± 0.95 vs 16.75 ± 0.82，pA/pF，$P<0.05$)(图 3-8)。

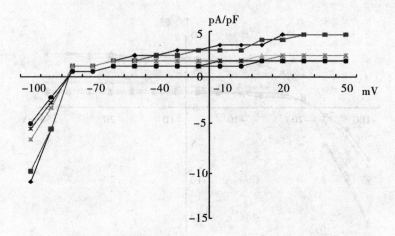

图 3-7 房颤组应用胺碘酮后：左心耳、右心耳、左心房、右心房、肺静脉和上腔静脉的 $I_{K,Ach}$ 电流 I-V 曲线。

$I_{K,Ach}$ 电流密度在左心耳和右心耳比右心房、左心房、肺静脉和上腔静脉高；左右心房没有差异。* $P<0.05$。(◆：右心耳细胞 ■：左心耳细胞 ▲：左心房细胞 ✕：右心房细胞 ✳：肺静脉细胞 ◆：上腔静脉细胞)

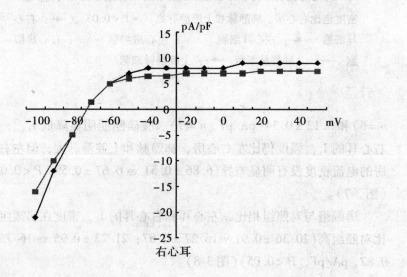

右心耳

第3章 胆碱能 M_2 受体和乙酰胆碱敏感钾通道在心房肌及其相邻大静脉的分布研究

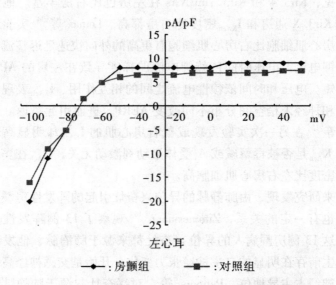

图 3-8 左右心耳的 $I_{K,Ach}$ 在房颤组和对照组的比较

左右心耳的 $I_{K,Ach}$ 电流密度在房颤组比对照组高，$P<0.05$。

讨 论

目前研究认为迷走神经刺激诱发房颤是由于引起心房内折返的发生，而这种折返是迷走神经刺激引起 AERP 和 APD 缩短及 AERP 和 APD 离散的直接原因[11]。Hirose[12]等观察灌注 Ach 和刺激迷走神经对房速诱发的影响，发现 Ach 和 VS 都升高极化恢复的离散，但是在相同的心房组织结构和起搏部位直接注射 Ach 却很少发现有传导阻滞发生，这可能与迷走神经及 M_2 受体在心房的分布不均有关。

有学者曾对 I_{KAch} 在心房的分布进行过研究。Sarmast 等[13]采用光学标测和双极记录观察绵羊诱发房颤的情况，其中优势频率和动态定量分别由光电信号和相位电影来判断，发现随着 Ach 浓度的增加，优势频率在左右心房升高，但在左房占主导，转子数量比右房也多见，Kir3.4 和 Kir3.1mRNAs 在左房也比右房丰富。他认为左房的 Kir3.X 通道和 I_{KAch} 密度比右房都高。Lomax 等[14]实验证实鼠的左房心肌细胞比右房心肌细胞有更高的外向快速延迟整流和内向整流钾电流。电压时间依赖钾电流的梯度导致在左房的 APD 比右房更短。电压和时间依赖性电流之间的相互作用、I_{KAch} 表现的不同水平和神经末梢空间分布不同改变 AERP，进而引起折返。但是 Lomax 等[15]在另一次实验发现成鼠右房心肌的 I_{KAch} 却明显高于左房，与 K_{Ach} 是否被毒蕈碱或 A_1 受体激动剂激动无关，I_{KAch} 在窦房结的电流密度比左右房心肌细胞高。

近来研究发现，由肺静脉的异位兴奋灶引起的阵发性房颤与迷走神经也有一定的关系，Zimmermann[16]观察了 13 例阵发性房颤病人，这 13 例房颤病人的异位兴奋灶都来源于肺静脉，他发现在房颤发生前存在明显的自主神经张力变化，开始是交感神经高，随后迷走神经占主导地位。Pappone 等[4]对兴奋灶起源于肺静脉的房颤病人进行消融时发现，同时在肺静脉口消融迷走神经比单独消融肺静脉病人的复发率明显降低。最近，Oral 等[17]对 188 例阵发性房颤病人进行肺静脉电隔离消融，依据病史分为迷走神经性房颤、肾上腺能房颤和随机发生的房颤，却发现肺静脉电隔离对迷走神经性房颤的治疗效果最低。Razavi[18]在对犬的肺静脉电隔离消融后发现左房的 AERP 对迷走神经刺激的反应性下降，房颤的易损性也明显降低。结果提示对肺静脉电隔离和去迷走神经消融治疗房颤，可能房颤的复发率下降不是肺静脉去迷走神经后的直接原因，而是因为肺静脉电隔离和去迷走神经后，导致迷走神经刺激对心房和心耳的影响下降的原因。

心脏的胆碱能受体主要为 M_2 受体，它与 Gk 和 Gi 两种 G 蛋白耦联，Gk 激活 K_{Ach}。K_{Ach} 又称为 Ach 调节钾通道，是一电导大门控过程快的钾通道，其活性需要有 Ca^{2+} 和 Mg^{2+} 参与，有内向整流特性[19]。目前研究认为 K_{Ach} 存在于心脏的窦房结、房室结、心房肌细胞，通过膜界间的通路可以激活 I_{KAch}，主要由 Ach 和 GTP 激活，也可超极化激活，其他配体例如腺苷和鞘胺醇磷酸脂接合百日咳毒敏感 G 联合受体也能激活 I_{KAch}。I_{KAch} 是 χ 亚基 Kir3.1/GIRK1

和 Kir3.4/GIRK4 的四聚物[20,21]，Gβγ 和组成钾通道的 χ 亚基可直接相互作用[22]。

为了探讨异位兴奋灶诱发房颤和迷走神经的关系，我们首次观察了 M_2 受体和 I_{KAch} 在肺静脉、上腔静脉、心耳和心房的分布情况，为消融迷走神经治疗房颤提供分子和离子通道基础。结果发现，在迷走神经刺激能诱发房颤的房颤组，M_2 受体和 I_{KAch} 在犬的肺静脉、上腔静脉、心耳和心房的分布存在明显差异，M_2 受体和 I_{KAch} 在心耳的电流密度最高，其次是左心房，而在右心房、肺静脉和上腔静脉的电流密度最低，I_{KAch} 的电流特性在上述部位没有明显差别；在迷走神经刺激未能诱发房颤的对照组，M_2 受体和 I_{KAch} 在心耳的电流密度也最高，在右心房、肺静脉和上腔静脉的电流密度最低，但心耳和左心房之间没有明显差别。结果提示迷走神经张力升高可能对肺静脉和上腔静脉的影响较小，而左右心房之间的 M_2 受体和 I_{KAch} 密度差别不是迷走神经刺激诱发房颤的主要原因，M_2 受体和 I_{KAch} 密度在左心耳和左心房的差异可能是迷走神经刺激诱发房颤的主要原因。

Sharifov[23] 在犬胆碱能房颤模型中发现在左心耳周围的折返显示一个慢的逐渐开始的短的 CL，随后以大约 60ms 的时间周期波动，另外，一个不同稳定折返是引导环，形成于左房游离壁和右心耳，在局灶型房颤的始发期，局灶激动可出现在左右心耳，靠近左房，并且随着 VS 强度增加而明显。结合本实验的结果，提示左右心耳在 VS 诱发房颤可能起到很重要的作用，心耳的微折返形成后，冲动向四周传导扩散，由于 VS 引起 APD 缩短并且离散升高，导致心房传导阻滞，引起一个或多的折返环，从而诱发房颤。

胺碘酮是治疗房颤较好的药物，研究认为，胺碘酮对 I_{KAch} 有抑制作用[24,25]，胺碘酮对腺苷引起 I_{KAch} 的阻断作用基本相似，说明胺碘酮主要作用 K_{Ach} 通道或 GTP 结合蛋白，而不是 M_2 受体。本实验也观察了胺碘酮对肺静脉、上腔静脉、心耳和心房 I_{KAch} 的影响。在房颤组，用 2mmol/L 胺碘酮后，肺静脉、上腔静脉、心耳和心房的 I_{KAch} 电流密度均减少，左右心房的 I_{KAch} 电流密度没有明显差别，但心耳的 I_{KAch} 电流密度仍然比左右心房高。结合我们的第二部分实验，胺碘酮虽能降低迷走神经刺激诱发房颤的发生率，但不能完全阻断迷走神经刺激的作用，可能与心耳和心房的I_{KAch}电流密度仍有差异有关。但胺碘酮不是一个选择性的通道阻断剂，它可以抑制I_{KAch}和几个内向电流（$I_{Ca,L}$）和外向电流（I_{Kr}，I_{Ks}，I_{Ki}）。KB130015是胺碘酮的衍生物，实验证实[26]通过直接作用细胞外的离子通道起到阻断I_{KAch}的作用，但它对心室肌的作用还不清楚，如果它具有选择性阻断I_{KAch}的作用，那么KB130015将是更有希望治疗迷走性房颤的药物。

结 论

M_2受体蛋白和I_{KAch}在心房肌的分布是不均一的，这种不均一可能是迷走神经刺激诱发折返和房颤的分子基础。心耳的分布明显高于其他部位，心耳可能在迷走神经诱发房颤中有重要作用。而肺静脉和上腔静脉在迷走性房颤的作用较小。胺碘酮可以阻断I_{KAch}并减少左右心房I_{KAch}大小的差异，此可能是其治疗胆碱能房颤的机制。

第4章 综述：迷走神经与心房颤动

赵庆彦　综　述
黄从新　审　校

心房颤动(房颤)是临床上常见的快速房性心律失常,在人群中发病率较高,并发症较多,疗效欠佳,故需要更深刻地认识房颤的发生机制。房颤的发生机制复杂,可能与多种因素有关,但最终房颤的维持可能是通过电重构。房颤电重构是指房颤引起心房电生理功能的改变,是心房对房颤节律的病理生理性适应[1],包括动作电位时程(APD)及心房有效不应期(AERP)缩短,APD及AERP的频率适应性降低,AERP离散度增加。基础和临床研究都已经证实使用乙酰胆碱(Acetylcholine,Ach)或刺激迷走神经可缩短AERP和心房激动的波长,增加AERP离散度,并能引发房颤的发生[2~4];阻断迷走神经或去心房的迷走神经可以阻止或降低房颤的发生[5]。下面就迷走神经与房颤关系的研究进展做一综述。

1. 心房的迷走神经支配

心脏副交感神经节前纤维由迷走神经背核和疑核发出,沿迷走神经心支行走,在心脏神经丛交换神经元后,分布于心脏。其中右侧迷走神经主要支配窦房结,左侧主要支配房室交界区[6~8]。心脏神经丛位于心外膜的脂肪结缔组织内,这些被心外膜脂肪结缔组织包绕的迷走神经丛又称心脏脂肪垫。Chiou等[9]根据迷走神经引起窦性心律减慢、房室结传导时间延长、AERP缩短的特性,通过对犬心房的不同部位射频消融,观察对这些指标的影响来确定消融部位是否分布迷走神经。他们发现上腔静脉和主动脉根部的中间脂肪垫是迷走神经主要分布区,比右肺动脉分布的迷走神经集中,这些迷走神经延伸到下腔静脉与左房之间的脂肪垫及右肺动脉的脂肪垫后到达左右心房,少数迷走神经纤维直接通过右肺动脉脂肪垫深入到心房肌,且迷走神经纤维在心房内的分布是不均一的。

在人类,与心房活动有关的脂肪垫分别位于右上和右下肺静脉的脂肪垫,及位于 Marshall 韧带心外膜附近、左上肺静脉和左下肺静脉的脂肪垫[10]。右上肺静脉的脂肪垫主要支配窦房结及附近心房肌,刺激该脂肪垫可以引起窦性心动过缓或窦性停搏,并使其支配区心房肌 AERP 缩短,而对房室结传导没有影响[11];右下肺静脉脂肪垫主要支配房室结及附近心房肌,刺激该脂肪垫可引起房室阻滞,并使其支配区心房肌 AERP 缩短,而对窦房结没有影响[12]。从脂肪垫发出的神经纤维如何支配心房肌及相互关系目前还不清楚,有研究表明人类左房神经纤维主要分布在心外膜,肺静脉口的神经纤维密度高于其远端部分,而心内膜仅有很细小的神经纤维分布[13]。

2. 迷走神经与房颤的关系

1972 年,Elsherif 等[14]就发现迷走神经对房颤的发生有重要作用,他通过压迫颈动脉窦诱发出了房颤或使心房扑动转为房颤。1978 年,Wilson 和 Davis[15]发现严重的恶心和呕吐可使房颤发作。Coumel 等[16]根据患者的房颤易在夜间和安静状态下发作,首先提出迷走神经房颤的概念。

另有临床研究也显示,心脏结构正常的阵发性房颤患者,迷走神经对房颤起始和维持都起重要作用[17-19],阵发性房颤患者在房颤发作前表现有自主神经张力的变化,即发作前数分钟先表现为交感神经张力的升高,随后出现迷走神经张力占优势[20,21],而且阵发性房颤起始时间也影响了自主神经在阵发性房颤起始和终止的张力[22]。Bertaglia 等对 25 例持续性房颤病人进行电转复后观察其心率变异性(HRV)的变化,48 小时内房颤再复发病人比没有复发病人的 LLF/HF 的比率明显低,他认为房颤在 48 小时内复发与房颤复律后迷走神经张力占有势有关[23]。

Vikman 等也对78例持续性房颤病人观察了电复律后HRV，随访一个月，有27例病人房颤复发，这些复发的病人，SDNN，InHF明显升高，InHR，InVLF明显降低，说明HF的升高反映了迷走神经张力增加，是房颤复律后再发的因素[24]。Vikman还对39例伴有器质性心脏病和孤立性房颤病人，通过心电图进行比较房颤发作前的心率紊度评估，结果显示房早后迷走神经张力短暂增强与房颤的发生有关[25]。Sutton等[26]对140例慢性房颤病人选择性直流电复律，也发现在复律前静脉注射阿托品消除高张力迷走神经后，病人更易恢复为窦性心律，说明高张力迷走神经可以阻止房颤终止。这均说明迷走神经过度兴奋可能与房颤密切相关。

动物实验也表明[27-29]，在给予颈胸迷走神经或心脏神经丛刺激时，对犬心房快速或期前刺激易诱发房颤。Sharifov等[30]在20只犬通过窦房结动脉灌注儿茶酚胺类或Ach及儿茶酚胺类和Ach混合物，比较诱发房颤的情况，发现异丙肾和肾上腺素（10～100 μmol/L）诱发房颤率分别为21%和17%，应用阿托品后可以阻止儿茶酚胺介导的房颤；Ach（2.8 +/-0.3 μmol/L）诱发房颤率是100%，普奈诺尔不能阻止Ach诱发的房颤，但能升高Ach诱发房颤的阈值，异丙肾能使Ach更易诱发房颤，结果说明虽然自主神经都能诱发房颤，胆碱能刺激在自发性房颤中起主要作用，肾上腺对胆碱能性房颤的诱发和维持起调节作用。Po等[31]把11只开胸犬分为两组，其中一组在脂肪垫注射Ach（1～10m mol/L），另一组注射卡巴可（1～10m mol/L）各0.5mL，发现2～5min后，有4只犬发生自发性房颤，另外7只犬用单一早搏刺激也很容易诱发出房颤。Ach组的房颤持续时间平均为10min，卡巴可组平均持续时间为38分钟，并在肺静脉与心房之间的脂肪垫观察到最短的房颤周长。他认为通过拟副交感神经的药注射到脂肪垫引起的急性自主神经重构很容易诱发房颤，自主神经节亢进对肺静脉诱发的局灶性房颤可能起关键作用。

但是，迷走神经在持续性房颤和永久性房颤中的作用还不清楚，Akyurek在慢性房颤病人发现HRV参数的抑制和迷走神经张力降低是房颤转复后复发的一个危险因素[32]。而且交感神经的作用也不能忽视，Lombardi 等[33]对110例阵发性房颤病人分析心率变异性后发现大部分阵发性房颤发作开始时交感神经占优势，而只有30%的阵发性房颤病人可以观察到迷走神经张力占优势。Berg 等[34]通过对73例阵发性房颤病人分析心率变异性认为，迷走性房颤并不是迷走神经反应性升高引起的，也没有直接证据说明迷走神经升高心脏的易损性，但迷走神经张力的升高与房颤的发生有关。

Kanoupakis 等[35]研究认为房颤复律后再复发是由于房颤时，心脏射血分数降低，使交感神经张力升高，迷走神经张力降低，窦性心律恢复后，心脏射血分数升高，使迷走神经张力过度恢复的原因。一般认为，心房的易损期位于 AERP 结束，相对不应期开始前，相当于心电图 QRS 波 R 波降支(或 S 波的后支)。因此需要提前的房性早搏(简称房早)落入该区方可诱发房颤。迷走神经可使心房肌细胞的 APD 和不应期缩短，并伴发房内兴奋传导的减弱。因此，不提前的房早也可诱发房颤，是房颤再发的主要原因。

3. 迷走神经对心房颤动电重构的影响

3.1 迷走神经与 AERP 的关系

迷走神经引起 AERP 缩短已被大多数学者认同[36~38]，迷走神经刺激缩短 AERP 和波长，并使心房短阵起搏诱发房颤的时间明显延长，使房颤更稳定。Jalife 等[39]实验刺激迷走神经或注射 Ach 可以使 AERP 明显缩短，同时房内传导发生障碍，这是引起房颤折返激动的电生理条件。Sharifov 等[40]也通过刺激迷走神经(10～50Hz)引发单个或多个房早和/或房颤，随着迷走神经刺激的加强，房早和房颤的发生增加，故他们认为随着刺激迷走神经频率的升高，房早和房颤的发生率增加。迷走神经刺激引起局部异位房早在心房内分布广泛，而一个单一的房早就足以引起房颤的发生。Schauerte 等[41]通过导管介入共标测7处心房不同位置的 AERP，在右肺动脉的部位刺激迷走神经，7个部位的 AERP 都明显缩短(123 ±4 vs 39 ±4ms)。后通过射频消融这些迷走神经都能使 AERP 明显延长(123 ±4 vs 127 ±3ms)，消融前电刺激迷走神经加心房程序刺激后伴随一个额外刺激可以使房颤很容易发生并可维持1h以上，消融迷走神经后，这种持续的房颤不再发生。在 Goette 等[42]动物模型的基础上，Takei 等[43]在快速心房刺激前先刺激迷走神经20min，发现快速刺激不能使 AERP 缩短。在右心房与右肺静脉连接处的脂肪组织用河豚毒素可以阻断迷走神经的"保护"作用。

房颤终止后或快速心房刺激终止后，迷走神经对电重构恢复期的 AERP 同样有重要作用。Blaauw 等[44]通过快速房室起搏终止后对电重构恢复期 AERP 的观察，发现 AERP 与迷走神经张力成反比关系，停止起搏后，AERP 逐渐延长，同时高张力迷走神经又使 AERP 缩短，故高张力迷走神经使 AERP 恢复时间明显延长。Miyauchi 等[45]对 15 例病人观察了短时快速心房起搏后自主神经阻断对 AERP 的影响，发现心房快速起搏终止后 3 分钟，阿托品组和阿托品加普奈诺尔组的 AERP 明显比对照组和普奈诺尔组长，而且AERP 恢复时间也明显缩短。结果说明副交感神经阻断能缩短快速心房起搏后 AERP 的恢复时间。

也有学者持不同观点，Wijffels 等[46]观察了房颤电重构出现前后阿托品与普奈洛尔对 AERP 的影响，结果表明在窦性心律与房颤维持 1～3d 时，阿托品与普奈洛尔对 AERP 只产生轻微影响。房颤引起的 AERP 缩短在使用阿托品和/或普奈洛尔后仍持续存在。慢性房颤时，使用阿托品和普奈洛尔，平均房颤间期虽也轻度延长（分别为 99±5，98±10ms），但与新近发生房颤时的房颤间期（148±13ms）相比却短得多。据此作者认为，交感和迷走神经张力增加是神经递质的高敏感性，而不是房颤诱导的 AERP 缩短的主要介导因素。Goette 等[42]通过对麻醉犬快速心房起搏（800 次/分）发现 AERP 下降大于 10%，电重构在起搏最初 30min 内发生很快，AERP 明显缩短（下降速度，为 24±2ms/h），之后 AERP 每小时仅缩短 1～2ms，但在快速起搏前阻断自主神经（使用阿托品与普奈洛尔），仍可看到 AERP 在最初 30min 明显缩短。他认为电重构恢复期高钙血症可延长 AERP 的恢复时间，说明 AERP 的变化与细胞内钙离子超载有关。Tieleman 等[47]也研究发现地高辛可明显延迟电重构恢复时间，看来影响房颤电重构的因素很多，迷走神经的影响还需进一步研究。

3.2 迷走神经与 AERP 离散度的关系

Gaspo 等[48]发现犬快速心房起搏 42d 后，AERP 离散度可明显升高，Blaauw 等[44]在 24h 快速心房刺激时未发现 AERP 离散度有明显变化，但发现刺激终止后 AERP 离散度明显升高（63±7.1 vs 44±4.2ms，$P=0.01$）。Liu 和 Nattel[49]通过刺激麻醉犬的交感神经和双迷走神经，发现交感神经和迷走神经对 AERP 有相似的影响，但刺激迷走神经可使房颤持续时间明显延长，并且使 AERP 离散度升高；而刺激交感神经对 AERP 的离散度影响不明显。Hirose 等[50]在研究垂体的腺苷酸环化酶多肽（PACAP）对犬心房电生理影响时发现，迷走神经刺激可使高位右心房的有效不应期（64±4.0ms）缩短，但对高位左心房（110±3.5ms）、低位左心房（102±11.5ms）、低位右心房 126±5.1ms）无明显影响。

临床上，Chen 等[51]对 50 例阵发性室上性心动过速病人（其中 23 例伴阵发性房颤、27 例不伴阵发性房颤）监测 AERP 离散度和 24h 心率变异性，结果显示伴有阵发性房颤的病人 AERP 基线比不伴阵发性房颤的病人高得多，并且 AERP 的离散度也明显升高，他认为心房电生理紊乱和迷走神经张力升高是 AERP 离散度升高的原因。以上资料说明，AERP 离散度升高是由于 AERP 恢复的空间分布不均一，并与迷走神经的分布不均一有密切关系[52]。由于迷走神经分布部位的 AERP 恢复延迟，使 AERP 离散度升高。Farch 等[53]认为心房空间分布的不同，AERP 也不同，AERP 变异性高，房颤的易损性与持续性与 AERP 或波长的关系不明显，而是与 AERP 的离散度有关，即 AERP 离散度升高是房颤发生的重要原因。

3.3 迷走神经与 APD 的关系

目前研究认为刺激迷走神经诱发房颤的原因是由于 APD 离散，导致折返的发生[54~57]，通过降低波长及增加多个折返环路发生的几率，从而使房颤的维持更稳定[58]。Hirose 等[59]在 12 例孤立犬右心房用高分析光标技术监测 APD，直接比较灌注 Ach 和刺激迷走神经对房速诱发的影响，发现 Ach 组的 APD 明显比迷走神经刺激组和对照组缩短，应用 Ach 后单一提前刺激很易引发房速，同样在迷走神经刺激组也有同样发现。与 Ach 组相比，迷走神经刺激组升高极化恢复的离散，与传导阻滞和不完全折返有关，但是在相同的心房组织结构和起搏部位直接注射 Ach 却很少发现有传导阻滞发生，这可能与迷走神经在心房的分布不均有关。所以刺激迷走神经诱发的房速不总是依赖极化恢复梯度。

交感和迷走神经都可以通过缩短 APD 诱发房颤，但与迷走神经相关的房颤比与交感神经相关的房颤更容易维持。Ashihara 等[60]利用计算机模拟，用 bidomain 离子通道模型构建同质的二维心肌片，发现交感神经的作用可以缩短 APD 并且使恢复坡度变平坦，这种结果可以导致旋波的产生并抑制旋波破裂，迷走神经释放的 Ach 也可以缩短 APD 和使恢复坡度变平坦，由于 I_{K1} 和 AERP 离散度的升高促使旋波的破裂，可以解释为什么交感神经相关的房颤持续时间短暂而与迷走神经相关的房颤持续时间长。Vigmond[61]在形态学上也用计算机模拟犬心房来探知 Ach 空间分布的不同对心律失常发生的作用，发现心房的结构能严格限制折返环的形成，波的分离仅仅发生在 APD 差别大的区域，认为 Ach 不均一产生的 APD 梯度的差别越大越能导致机化激动的破裂。赵庆彦等对在体犬迷走神经刺激观察对 APD 影响和诱发房颤的情况，认为 APD 缩短是迷走神经刺激诱发折返和房颤的基础，而单独心房肌 APD 离散升高不是房颤诱发的主要原因，APD 离散度和 APD 的比值对评价诱发房颤的情况[62]可能更好。

当然，交感神经和迷走神经相互影响对心房肌的作用也很重要，他们对心房的影响有协同作用，虽然有研究表明在犬交感神经刺激诱发房颤起的作用较小[63]，但 Olgin[64]研究表明阶段性去交感神经可导致去神经区域内的心房 ERP 缩短，ERP 的离散度升高，在没有迷走神经刺激情况下，可增加诱发房颤的几率。Patterson 等[65]对正常犬离体肺静脉采用电刺激自主神经发现，同时刺激交感神经和迷走神经可缩短肺静脉积袖 APD，诱发肺静脉局灶性冲动，阿托品和阿替洛尔都能有效地抑制这些局灶性冲动的发生。不容忽视的是三磷酸腺苷（ATP）也存在于交感神经和迷走神经末梢，当刺激神经时能随着去甲肾上腺素和 Ach 共同释放。Hara 等[66]就发现细胞外 ATP 对豚鼠心房细胞的 I_{KAch} 有双重影响，交感神经和迷走神经对心房的协同作用是否与此有关还需进一步研究。

虽然迷走神经对房颤电重构的影响机制不十分明了，但迷走神经对房颤电重构的重要作用已被大多数学者所认同。有学者报道，心房电重构在心房扑动时也可见到，看来，心房电重构并非房颤所独有。是心房电重构为因，房颤为果？还是房颤为因，心房电重构为果？其因果关系尚不清楚。目前大多数学者的研究都是观察急性心房起搏情况下的电重构与迷走神经的关系，而其远期情况还需进一步研究。引起房颤电重构的原因不仅是迷走神经，还有细胞内钙离子超载等原因，迷走神经与其他因素的关系如何？心动过速导致迷走神经活动的变化是由于心室率的增加还是房性心动过速，还需进一步研究。

4. 迷走神经对心房颤动影响的离子通道基础

4.1 胆碱能 M 受体和 Ach 激活钾通道的结构和功能

迷走神经末梢释放 Ach 与心肌细胞膜上的胆碱能 M_2 受体结合，激活 K_{Ach}，促进 K^+ 外流并使膜超极化[67]。对 I_K，I_f，I_{Ca} 均产生抑制效应，使 3 期复极加速和舒张期超极化，增大舒张期电位与阈电位距离。Ach 还直接抑制钙通道，减慢 4 期自动除极速率，使自律性降低。

心脏的胆碱能受体主要为 M_2 受体，目前证实的其他亚型还有 M_1、M_3、M_4 和 M_5 亚型，有研究认为 M_3 和 M_4 受体激活的 I_{KM3} 和 I_{K4AP} 也与 APD 缩短和房颤的诱发有关[68~70]。研究最多的还是 M_2 受体，它与 Gk 和 Gi 两种 G 蛋白耦联，Gk 激活心房毒蕈碱激活钾通道(atrial muscainic-activated K channels, K_{Ach})；Gi 抑制受体-腺苷酸环化酶(AC)的活性，减少 cAMP 生成，降低蛋白激酶 A(PKA)活性，关闭 L 型钙通道，开放 KV 电压依赖性钾通道(KDR)。上述两种钾通道开放均产生复极化电流，增加舒张电位而导致负性频率作用。K_{Ach} 又称 Ach 调节钾通道，是一电导大门控过程快的钾通道，其活性需要有[Ca^{2+}]和[Mg^{2+}]参与，有内向整流特性。K_{Ach} 存在于心脏的窦房结、房室结、心房肌细胞，通过膜界间的通路可以激

活 I_{KAch}，主要由 Ach 和 GTP 激活，也可超极化激活，其他配体例如腺苷和鞘胺醇磷酸脂结合百日咳毒敏感 G 联合受体也能激活 I_{KAch}[71]。I_{KAch} 是 χ 亚基 Kir3.1/GIRK1 和 Kir3.4/GIRK4 的四聚物[72,73]，Gβγ 和组成钾通道的 χ 亚基可直接相互作用[74]。在细胞表达系统中，GIRK1 和 GIRK4 都与 I_{KAch} 的特性有关，如果缺乏 GIRK4，GIRK1 也不能形成有功能的离子通道。Bettahi 等[75]发现在击昏小鼠心房肌细胞 Kir3.1 的降低不影响 Kir3.4 蛋白水平，但可以降低卡巴可（Carbachol，Cch）引起的 I_{KAch}，他认为 K_{Ach} 的特性主要与 Kir3.1 有关，Kir3.1 可增加 K_{Ach} 通道的活性。

4.2 K_{Ach} 在心房的分布

心房内神经支配的不均一是迷走神经刺激导致房颤的重要原因，Sarmast 等[76]采用光学标测和双极记录观察绵羊诱发房颤的情况，其中优势频率和动态定量分别由光电信号和相位电影来判断，发现随着 Ach 浓度的增加，优势频率在左右心房升高，但在左房占主导，转子数量比右房也多见，Kir3.4 和 Kir3.1mRNAs 在左房也比右房丰富。他认为左房的 Kir3.X 通道和 I_{KAch} 密度比右房都高。Lomax 等[77]实验证实鼠的左房心肌细胞比右房心肌细胞有更高的外向快速延迟整流和内向整流钾电流。电压时间依赖钾电流的梯度导致在左房的 APD 比右房更短。电压和时间依赖性电流之间的相互作用、I_{KAch} 表现的不同水平和神经末梢空间分布不同改变 AERP，进而引起折返。但是 Lomax 等[78]在另一次实验发现成鼠右房心肌的 I_{KAch} 却明显高于左房，与 K_{Ach} 是否被毒蕈碱或 A_1 受体激动剂激动无关，I_{KAch} 在窦房结的电流密度比左右房心肌细胞高。

黄从新等对犬心房肌及其相邻大静脉的 K_{Ach} 研究发现，K_{Ach} 在左右心耳分布最高，其次是左右心房，左心房的 K_{Ach} 分布比右心房高，而肺静脉和上腔静脉的分布最少，他认为在迷走神经刺激导致心房内折返和诱发房颤过程中，心耳可能起到重要的作用[79]。

4.3 毒蕈碱受体激动剂对 K_{Ach} 的影响

研究证明通过对副交感神经末梢在心房不同部位的刺激释放 Ach 所引起的 AERP 离散足以导致折返，并且静注或灌注 Ach 或腺苷都能引发房性心动过速（房速）和房颤的发生[80,81]。但如果心房内缺少 Ach 不能诱发房颤的发生[80]。

Ach 通过激活百日咳毒敏感 G 蛋白促进心肌 K^+ 外流已经被证实，$G\chi$ 和 $G\beta$ 亚基的活性对不同酶和离子通道有多种反应，包括电压时间依赖性钙通道和 G 蛋白门控 K_{Ach}[81]，房速通常由心房肌折返激动引起，这种折返是由于心房组织不应期的非均一性，电压时间依赖性钠电流(I_{Na})和 G 蛋白门控 I_{KAch} 的失活是心肌不应期的基础。在膜电位超极化 I_{Na} 快速恢复，时程与 APD 和膜静息电位（RMP）的时程有关，近来发现电压时间依赖性钾通道异种基因的表达影响左房和右房的 AP 除极和静息膜电位[76,82]。这种异质性引起不应期的离散和心房折返[83,84]。Zou 等[85]在不同 Ach 浓度情况下，用二维犬心房数学模式来模拟胆碱能房颤，发现单一优势转子或多发折返旋子都能维持颤动，并与不同基质大小有关。

有研究认为 I_{KAch} 电流密度在鼠心房有倾斜度，并不依赖钾离子电流是否被毒蕈碱受体激活，因为腺苷依赖性钾电流的倾斜度也可观察到。Lomax 等[78]研究认为毒蕈碱受体信号不单包括 K_{Ach}，也可以通过 $G\alpha$ 亚基降低细胞内 cAMP 聚集，$G\alpha$ 亚基调节多个膜传导包括电压时间依赖性钙电流。Cch 对钾电流和 AP 的作用能被毒蕈碱受体拮抗剂阻断，毒蕈碱激动剂和 A_1 激动剂对 K_{Ach} 的影响基本一样，K_{Ach} 能被几个百日咳毒敏感 G 联合受体激活，包括 Edg-3、A_1 和毒蕈碱受体，K_{Ach} 的激活对心房肌细胞的 RMP 有明显的超极化作用，并且心房肌细胞灌注 Cch 可以引起 APD 明显缩短。

Ach 不仅对 I_{KAch} 有影响，Wang 等[86]发现在猫心房肌 Ach 的减少能改变膜电位、升高 $I_{Ca,L}$ 的钙离子流，并引起肌质网细胞内钙离子超载，导致心房肌细胞的延迟后除极。这一现象是由于 Ach 的减少引起 cAMP 依赖 PKA 通道的反跳刺激，在心室肌和心室浦肯野纤维也被观察到。但猫的心房肌细胞表现明显的内源性和 cAMP 活性的依赖性，不需要 β 肾上腺能的刺激作用。但是 Gi 蛋白对 cAMP-PKA 信号通路的抑制是 Ach 抑制 $I_{Ca,L}$ 的钙内流的主要机制。

4.4 K_{Ach} 在房颤中重构的研究

Shi 等[87]对充血性心力衰竭（CHF）的犬诱发房颤，观察三种 Ach 受体亚基的不同改变，发现 I_{KAch} 和延缓性整流钾电流 I_{K4AP}（4-

aminopyridine，M4 受体激活)的电流密度分别降低 45% 和 55%，延缓性整流钾电流 I_{KM3}(M3 受体激活)的电流密度升高 75%。Western blot 分析也显示 M_2 和 M_4 亚基的受体密度分别下降 33% 和 22%，而 M_3 亚基的受体密度升高 2.3 倍。他认为在 CHF 导致房颤的电重构中，这主要是因为多种 Ach 受体亚基的不同改变导致所耦联的钾离子通道变化的结果。Dobrev 等[88]对慢性房颤病人心房组织 Kir2.1 和 GIRK4 定量分析发现 I_{K1} 转录上调，而 I_{KAch} 下调，并且 K_{Ach} 通道亚基表达也降低。与 I_{K1} 转录上调相对应，单个心肌细胞和肌小梁的静息膜电位负值加大，并且减弱毒蕈碱受体对 APD 的缩短作用。可能是心房肌细胞通过下调 K_{Ach} 来对抗心房有效不应期的缩短，阻止电重构，是心房肌细胞对长期快心率的一种适应。最近，Dobrev 等[89]对慢性房颤病人和窦性心律病人心房肌细胞观察 $I_{K,Ach}$ 的选择性阻断剂 tertiapin 对 $I_{K,Ach}$ 的阻断作用，发现在慢性房颤心房肌细胞比窦性心律心房肌细胞浓度依赖性高，在单通道膜片钳记录中，发现 $I_{K,Ach}$ 活性在慢性房颤心房肌细胞比窦性心律心房肌细胞大，结果说明虽然在慢性房颤病人心房肌细胞的 K_{Ach} 下调，但其单通道 $I_{K,Ach}$ 开放率却增加了。

4.5 药物对 I_{KAch} 和房颤的影响

胺碘酮是治疗房颤较好的药物，研究认为胺碘酮对 Cch、腺苷和 GTP-γ-S 引起 I_{KAch} 的阻断作用基本相似，说明胺碘酮主要作用 K_{Ach} 通道或 GTP 结合蛋白，而不是 M_2 受体[90-92]，但胺碘酮不是一个选择性的通道阻断剂，它可以抑制 I_{KAch} 和几个内向电流($I_{Ca,L}$)和外向电流(I_{Kr}，I_{Ks}，I_{Ki})。黄从新等[79]观察胺碘酮对犬左右心房 I_{KAch} 电流密度时发现，左心房的 I_{KAch} 明显比右心房高，电流都表现出强的内向整流性，用 2m mol/L 胺碘酮后，左右心房的 I_{KAch} 明显减少。左右心房减少后的 I_{KAch} 电流密度没有差异，说明相同浓度的胺碘酮对 I_{KAch} 电流大的作用相对强，对左右心房 I_{KAch} 阻断后使 I_{KAch} 的差异降低，电流的趋于一致降低了折返的发生率。决萘达隆(dronedarone)的分子结构和胺碘酮相近，Guillemare 等[93]研究决萘达隆对 K_{Ach} 通道的影响，发现在同样的浓度范围都可以阻滞 GTP-γ-S 和 Cch 引起的钾电流，决萘达隆的阻断作用比胺碘酮约高

100倍，也是主要作用Ach敏感性钾通道或GTP结合蛋白，而不是M_2受体。KB130015是胺碘酮的衍生物，实验也证实[94]通过直接作用细胞外的离子通道起到阻断I_{KAch}的作用，但它对心室肌的作用还不清楚，如果它具有选择性阻断I_{KAch}的作用，那么KB130015将是有希望治疗迷走性房颤的药物。

Watanabe等[95]研究丙吡胺(disopyramide)对离体豚鼠心房肌细胞的影响发现丙吡胺是通过阻断毒蕈碱受体，进而抑制I_{KAch}，并且可以逆转Cch对AERP的缩短作用。Sugiura[96]等对犬进行迷走神经刺激，也观察丙吡胺对心房肌电生理的影响，发现应用丙吡胺后HRV的HF明显降低，并且也明显降低迷走神经刺激增强HF的效应(from +492% to +127%)，用丙吡胺后，迷走神经刺激不能诱发房颤。但pilsicainide却没有明显的影响。Fedorov[97]等对6只开胸犬迷走神经刺激诱发房颤，静脉应用RG-2(5mg，10mg，20mg，40mg/kg)，发现RG-2在迷走神经刺激前后都能升高AERP，并有剂量依赖性，但不能改变传导速率。5 mg/kg能终止4只犬的房颤，但不能阻止房颤的再诱发，20 mg/kg和40 mg/kg能完全终止房颤诱发。心外膜激动图也显示RG-2能降低微波数量，房颤终止前房颤周长也明显升高，可能与RG-2升高AERP有关。

Hara等[98]研究发现chloroquine，primaquine，pyrimethamine和quinidine都能阻断卡巴可激活的I_{KAch}，这些药物也对细胞内GT-PgammaS激活I_{KAch}有阻断作用，说明抗疟药可以通过不同分子机制产生抗胆碱能作用。索他洛尔(sotalol)是一强效非心脏选择性β受体阻滞药，兼有III类抗心律失常药特性，研究发现索他诺尔不但对I_{KAch}有阻断作用，而且对I_{KM3}也有阻断作用。但这些药物都不是治疗房颤的理想药物，如果我们发现一种选择性阻断K_{Ach}的药物将是药物治疗房颤的一大进步，因为K_{Ach}不参与心室的复极，所以不会引起如尖端扭转性室速的恶性心律失常。

5. 心脏迷走神经消融在房颤中的作用

5.1 心脏神经消融治疗房颤的基础研究

Randall[99,100]等在犬心房外膜首先对其脂肪垫进行外科手术切除而去神经治疗,认为选择性去神经治疗是可行的。Chiou[9]等应用射频消融方法对心外膜脂肪垫位点进行消融,结果发现消融心外膜脂肪垫可以消除迷走神经介导的心房ERP缩短及在迷走神经刺激下房颤的诱发。Elvan[101]等报道应用类似外科迷宫手术的方法,对犬正常心脏实施心外膜线性射频消融,结果发现犬心房射频消融能减少房颤的诱发和持续时间。尽管当时可能没有消融心脏脂肪垫或神经丛的概念,但其资料提示这些损伤效应实际上类似脂肪垫消融,其损伤线路包括右房后中部上下腔静脉之间,以及紧邻第三脂肪垫下方的线路。这些损伤可以阻断脂肪垫向其所支配区域心房肌的神经放射,所以可以显著减轻左右心房迷走神经介导的ERP缩短及房颤的诱发。研究同时表明仅仅局限于左房的线性损伤也能消除迷走神经刺激时房颤的诱发。但Hirose[102]等仅仅针对支配窦房结及其附近右房肌的脂肪垫实施消融,即右房部分去迷走神经,尽管消融后右房ERP增加,但反而增加了房颤的诱发率。作者诱发房颤的方法是在双侧迷走神经干刺激的同时,也对左房进行电刺激,由于右房迷走神经去除,而左房迷走神经支配还存在,当双侧迷走神经刺激时,既可导致左右心房显著的复极电位差,更易诱发房颤。因此,右房选择性去自主神经支配将显著增加左右心房之间ERP的离散度,增加房颤诱发率,所以针对心房完全去迷走神经治疗可能有效地减少房颤发作。

以上方法均通过开胸实施心外膜消融,近年来有学者通过经皮血管径路心内膜导管消融的方法,同样可以消融位于心外膜的脂肪垫。Schauerte[41]等的研究对象是11只犬,对其中7只犬采用经外周血管径路沿着右肺静脉对第三脂肪垫进行射频消融,其中2只犬附加下腔静脉(支配房室结脂肪垫)消融,1只犬附加上腔静脉(支配窦房结脂肪垫)消融,结果显示,射频消融后能消除迷走神经刺激状态下所有部位心房ERP的缩短及其离散度的增加,消融前在迷走神经刺激状态下能诱发的房颤不能再诱发。作者认为,经血管射频消融改良心房迷走神经系统能消除迷走神经介导的房颤,并能为进一步评价动物慢性房颤模型及最终实施人类迷走性房颤的射频消融提供新途径。便于能更准确地在心内膜对其他脂肪垫进行定位和消融，该研究组在另一项研究中先通过开胸在8只犬心外膜直视定位左右上肺静脉脂肪垫并将刺激电极缝合于脂肪垫，然后关闭胸腔，再通过外周血管径路行房间隔穿刺将Lasso电极送至左右上肺静脉开口附近，结果所有犬脂肪垫通过心内膜与心外膜电极刺激方法均得到确认，并在其中7只犬中，于右房间隔附近的右上肺静脉处也能确认脂肪垫的存在，实施射频消融后，术前能诱发房颤的7只犬，术后仅1只犬能再次诱发房颤，而且所有犬心房ERP不再呈现迷走神经刺激所造成的缩短[103]。

Razavi[104]在对犬的肺静脉电隔离消融后发现左房的AERP对迷走神经刺激的反应性下降，房颤的易损性也明显降低。结果提示对肺静脉电隔离和去迷走神经消融治疗房颤，可能房颤的复发率下降不是肺静脉去迷走神经后的直接原因，而是因为肺静脉电隔离和去迷走神经后，导致迷走神经刺激对心房和心耳的影响下降的原因。

5.2 心脏神经消融治疗房颤的临床研究

Scherlag[10]等比较了33例接受常规消融治疗＋脂肪垫消融（联合治疗）与27例单纯接受常规消融治疗（常规治疗组）的房颤患者的疗效。常规消融是指完全的左右肺静脉前庭的隔离，如果隔离后仍能诱发房性心动过速，再附加线性消融或局灶消融。两组阵发性房颤分别为17和14例，持续性房颤分别为16与13例。脂肪垫消融前，先对与4根肺静脉相关的脂肪垫进行确认，即通过导管在心内膜相应部位实施高频电刺激，如果呈现阳性迷走反应，提示刺激点位于脂肪垫，阳性迷走反应是指高频电刺激开始数秒内窦性心率减慢或停搏，或房颤时平均RR间期延长至少50％以上，而当刺激终止后数秒内心率即可恢复至刺激前状态。脂肪垫消融的范围包括所有对高频电刺激呈阳性迷走反应的位点。消融终点是所有位点的阳性迷走反应消失。结果显示，单纯进行脂肪垫消融即可消除95％患者肺静脉的触发灶，但不能减少持续房颤的诱发率，附加肺静脉前庭隔离后，所有患者肺静脉触发灶均被消除。联合治疗组与常规治疗组手术结束即刻，持续性房颤的诱发分别为24％和26％，二者之间并无显著差异。但对联合治疗组平均5个月和常规治疗组平均12个月的随访发现,联合治疗组91%的患者无房颤发作,包括所有17例阵发性房颤和13例持续性房颤;常规治疗组无房颤发作者仅70%,包括10例阵发性房颤和9例持续性房颤。而且脂肪垫消融放电次数明显少于肺静脉前庭隔离治疗,不存在导致肺静脉狭窄的可能性,形成血栓栓塞的风险也很小,初步显示了脂肪垫消融的潜在优势。

Platt[105]等报道了26例持续性或慢性房颤患者单纯接受脂肪垫射频消融的临床结果,通过外周血管径路穿刺房间隔将lasso电极置入左房,在肺静脉前庭部位寻找并确定消融位点,用于确定脂肪垫的高频电刺激频率为20Hz,脉宽0.1ms,电压12V。消融参数为功率35W,温度55℃,时间120s。结果表明,每个脂肪垫平均消融4次,即刻手术成功率89%,对于所有呈迷走阳性反应的脂肪垫均接受消融者,其即刻手术成功率为96%。无早期复发和肺静脉狭窄。22例即刻成功病例中,14例仍需服用抗心律失常药物(手术前无效),8例不需要任何药物即可维持窦性心律。平均随访6个月仍有84%的患者维持窦性心律。

已经证明去迷走神经能提高环肺静脉消融的效果,在阵发性和慢性房颤都有很高的成功率[106]。Pappone[5]等在对房颤行射频消融时,297例患者在接受环肺静脉消融过程中,发现34%的患者,左房内某些位点对高能量射频电流产生显著心动过缓等迷走反应,针对这些位点继续消融可使迷走反应消失。经过12个月的随访,术中有迷走反应的患者99%无房颤复发,而术中没有迷走反应的患者仅有74%患者无房颤复发。而这些位点恰好与Scherlag等研究中对高频电刺激呈现阳性迷走反应的位点类似,或者说,Pappone等消融的位点可能就是与心外膜脂肪垫相对应的心内膜区域,实际上是在心内膜对心外膜脂肪垫实施了射频消融。

Takahashi[107]等对25例房颤病人(18例阵发性房颤,7例慢性房颤)观察后发现,迷走神经刺激时颤动周长在冠状窦和肺静脉明显降低,在房室传导恢复后都能恢复到基线,颤动周长的缩短在肺静脉发生较早且更明显,这种作用首先出现在肺静脉,随后出现在肺静脉口和冠状窦,他认为迷走神经刺激与房颤周长的缩短有关,迷走神经刺激增强了肺静脉的驱动效应。最近，Oral[108]等对188例阵发性房颤病人进行肺静脉电隔离消融，依据病史分为迷走神经性房颤、肾上腺能房颤和随机发生的房颤，却发现肺静脉电隔离对迷走神经性房颤的治疗效果最低。

从目前的研究结果来看，不论是基础研究还是临床治疗，主要是针对心脏迷走神经丛的消融，这种选择性心房去迷走神经在短时期表现有抗心律失常的作用。但去迷走神经的长期安全性还需进一步观察，曾有报道射频消融前、中、后间隔可损伤节前或节后迷走神经纤维，继而产生不适当窦性心动过速[109]，此外在动物实验中脂肪垫的射频消融还可损害心率变异性和压力反射的敏感性，尤其对于老年人和心室功能异常情况下，而且心外膜消融或对下腔静脉和右肺静脉间的迷走神经脂肪垫消融，增加了室性心律失常的危险性[110]。房颤的外科手术或消融治疗都是对迷走神经区域性和选择性的，而对心房、窦房结、房室结的交感神经没有影响，所以交感神经对心率的影响仍存在[111~113]。Hirose[102]研究认为部分去迷走神经，尤其对右心房去迷走神经，反而增加了房颤的易损性。并且动物模型实验结果不能推广到人类，Cumming等[114]报道对包含迷走神经节的前脂肪垫保留后，反而能降低手术后房颤的发生。因此，心房的去神经治疗可能导致自主神经张力调节失衡；其次是目前神经消融很难做到完全去神经化，而且去神经化到何种程度即可治愈房颤也不清楚，心脏是否存在迷走神经再生的问题也不明了。另有报道致心律失常是由于神经损害后，交感神经和副交感神经轴突再生和神经芽植产生区域差别的原因[115-117]。所以，区域性去迷走神经的有效性和安全性需要在实验研究和临床研究做全面的评估。

参考文献

引言

[1] Prystowsky EN, Benson JD, Woodrow MD, et al. Management of patients with atrial fibrillation: a statement for healthcare professionals from the subcommittee on electrocardiography and electrophysiology, American Heart Association. Circulation, 1996, 93: 1262-1277.

[2] Liu J, Huang CX, Bao MW, et al. Ectopic activity induced by atrial pressure in rabbit pulmonary vein in vitro. Chin Med J, 2005, 118: 1210-1213.

[3] Jais P, Haissaguerre M, Shah DC, et al. A focal source of atrial fibrillation treated by discrete radiofrequency ablation. Circulation, 1997, 95: 572-576.

[4] Haissaguerre M, Shah DC, Jais P, et al. Electrophysiological breakthroughs from the left atrium to the pulmonary veins. Circulation, 2000, 102: 2463-2465.

[5] Haissaguerre M, Jais P, Shah DC, et al. Spontaneous initiation of atrial fibrillation by ectopic beats originating in the pulmonary veins. N Engl J Med, 1998, 339: 659-666.

[6] 王晞，黄从新，江洪，等. 兔肺静脉心肌袖组织学特性研究. 中华心律失常学杂志, 2003, 7(4): 241-243.

[7] Tsai CF, Tai CT, Hsieh MH, et al. Initiation of atrial fibrillation by ectopic beats originating from the superior vena cava: electrophysiological characteristics and results of radiofrequency ablation. Circu-

lation, 2000, 102: 67-74.

[8] Goya M, Ouyang F, Ernst S, et al. Electroanatomic mapping and catheter ablation of break-throughs from the right atrium to the superior vena cava in patients with atrial fibrillation[J]. Circulation, 2002, 106: 1317-1320.

[9] 谢双伦,黄从新,江洪,等. 兔上下腔静脉中的心肌细胞组织结构研究. 中华心律失常学杂志, 2003, 7: 234-237.

[10] Jalife J. Rotors and spiral waves in atrial fibrillation. J Cardiovasc Electrophysiol. 2003, 14: 776-780.

[11] Wijfells MC, Kirchhof CJ, Dorland R, et al. Atrial fibrillation begets atrial fibrillation. A study in awade chronically instrumented goats. Circulation, 1995, 92: 1954-1968.

[12] Danshi M, Melnyk P, Gaspo R, et al. Ionic mechanisms of electrical remodeling in human atrial fibrillation. Cardiovase Res, 2003, 84: 776-784.

[13] Ramdat Missier AR, Opthof T, Van Hemel NM, et al. Increased dispersion of refractoriness in patients with idiopathic paroxysmal atrial fibrillation. J Am Coll Cardiol, 1992, 19: 1531-1535.

[14] Cosio FG, Palacias J, Vidal JM, et al. Electrophysiological studies in atrial fibrillation. Slow conduction of premature impulses: a possible manifestation of the background for reentry. Am J Cardiol, 1983, 51: 122-130.

[15] Schauerte P, Scherlag BJ, Patterson E, et al. Focal atrial fibrillation: Experimental evidence for a pathophysiologic role of the autonomic nervous system. J Cardiovasc Electrophysiol, 2001, 12: 592-599.

[16] Pappone C, Santinelli V, Manguso F, et al. Pulmonary vein denervation enhances long-term benefit after circumferential ablation for paroxysmal atrial fibrillation. Circulation, 2004, 109: 327-334.

[17] Coumel P. Autonomic influences in atrial tachyarrhythmias. J Cardiovasc Electrophysiol, 1996, 7: 999-1007.

[18] Chen YJ, Chen SA, Tai CT, et al. : Role of atrial electrophysiology and autonomic nervous system in patients with supraventricular tachycardia and paroxysmal atrial fibrillation. J Am Coll Cardiol 1998, 32: 732-738.

[19] Singh J, Mela T, Ruskin J. Sleep (vagal)-induced atrial fibrillation. Circulation, 2004; 110: 32-33.

[20] Bettoni M, Zimmermann M. Autonomic tone variations before the onset of paroxysmal atrial fibrillation [J]. Circulation, 2002, 105: 2753-2759.

[21] Fioranelli M, Piccoli M, Mileto GM, et al. Analysis of heart rate variability five minutes before the onset of paroxysmal atrial fibrillation[J]. PACE, 1999; 22: 743-749.

[22] Tomita T, Takei M, Saikawa Y, et al. Role of autonomic tone in the initiation and termination of paroxysmal atrial fibrillation in patients without structural heart disease. J Cardiovasc Electrophysiol, 2003, 14: 565-566.

[23] Bertaglia E, Zoppo F, Bonanno C, et al. Autonomic modulation of the sinus node following electrical cardioversion of persistent atrial fibrillation: relation with early recurrence. In J Cardiol, 2005, 102: 219-23.

[24] Schauerte P, Scherlag BJ, Pitha J, et al. Catheter ablation of cardiac autonomic nerves for prevention of vagal atrial fibrillation[J]. Circulation, 2000, 102: 2774-2780.

[25] Oral H, Chugh A, Scharf C, et al. Pulmonary vein isolation for vagotonic, adrenergic, and random episodes of paroxysmal atrial fibrillation. J Cardiovasc Electrophysiol, 2004, 15: 402-406.

[26] Razavi M, Zhang S, Yang D, et al. Effects of pulmonary vein ablation on regional atrial vagal innervation and vulnerability to atrial fibrillation in dogs. J Cardiovasc Electrophysiol, 2005, 16: 879-884.

[27] Sarmast F, Kolli A, Zaitsev A, et al. Cholinergic atrial fibrilla-

tion: I_{KAch} gradients determine unequal left/right atrial frequencies and rotor dynamics. Cardiovasc Res, 2003, 59: 863-873.

[28] Lomax AE, Kondo CS, Giles WR. et al. Comparison of time-and voltage-dependent K^+ currents in myocytes from left and right atria of adult mice[J]. Am J Physiol Heart Circ Physiol, 2003, 285: H1837-1848.

[29] Lomax AE, Rose RA, Giles WR. et al. Electrophysiological evidence for a gradient of G protein-gated K^+ current in adult mouse atria. Br J Pharmacol, 2003, 140: 576-584.

第1章

[1] Wijffels Mc, Kirchhof CJ, Dorland R, et al. Atrial fibrillation beget-atrial fibrillation: a study in awake chronically in strumented goats. Circulation 92: 1954, 1995

[2] Takei M, Tsuboi M, Usui T, et al: Vagal stimulation prior to atrial rapid pacing protects the atrium from electrical remodeling in anesthetiaed dogs. Jpn Circ J 65: 1077, 2001

[3] Coumel P. Neurogenic and humoral influences of the autonomic nervous system in the determination of paroxysmal atrial fibrillation. Mount Kisco, N Y: Futura Publishing Co, 1989, 213-232.

[4] Chen YJ, Chen SA, Tai CT, et al. Role of atrial electrophysiology and autonomic nervous system in patients with superventricular tachycardia and paroxysmal atrial fibrillation[J]. J Am Coll Cardiol, 1998, 32(3): 732-737.

[5] Blaauw Y, Tieleman RG, Brouwer J, et al: Tachycardia induced electrical remodeling of the atria and the autonomic nervous system in goats. PACE 1999, 22: 1656-1667.

[6] Sutton AG, Khurana C, Hall JA, et al. The use of atropine for facilitation of direct current cardioversion from atrial fibrillation-results of a pilot study. Clin Cardiol, 1999, 22: 712-714.

[7] Chen YJ, Chen SA, Tai CT, et al: Role of atrial electrophysiology

and autonomic nervous system in patients with supraventricular tachycardia and paroxysmal atrial fibrillation. J Am Coll Cardiol, 1998, 32: 732-738.

[8] Jose AD, Taylor RR: Automatic blockade by Propranolol and Atropine to study intrinsic myocardial function in man. J Clin Invest, 1969, 48: 2019-2031.

[9] Suttorp MJ, Kingma JH, Lie-A-Huen L, Mast EG: Intravenous flecainide versus verapamil for acute conversion of paroxysmal atrial fibrillation or flutter to sinus rhythm. Am J Cardiol, 1989, 63: 693696.

[10] Van Gelder IC, Crijins HJ, Van Gilst WH, Verwer R, Lie KI: Prediction of sinus rhythm from direct-current electrical cardioversion of chronic atrial fibrillation and flutter. Am J Cardiol, 1991, 68: 41-46.

[11] Jalife J, Berenfeld O, Skanes A. et al. Mechanisms of atrial fibrillation: mother rotors or multiple daughter wavelets, or both [J]? J Cardiovasc Electrophysiol, 1998, 9: S2-12.

[12] Sharifov OF, Zaitsev AV, Rosenshtraukh LV, et al. Spatial distribution and frequency dependence of arrhythmogenic vagal effects in canine atria [J]. J Cardiovasc Electrophysiol, 2000, 11: 1029-1042.

[13] Schauerte P, Scherlag BJ, Pitha J, Scherlag MA, Reynolds D, et al: Catheter ablation of cardiac autonomic nervous for prevention of vagal atrial fibrillation. Circullation 102: 2774, 2000.

[14] Wijffels MC, Kirchhof CJ, Dorland R, et al. Electrical remodeling due to atrial fibrillation in chronically instrumented conscious goats: roles of neurohumoral changes, ischemia, atrial stretch, and high rate of electrical activation [J]. Circulation, 1997, 96: 3710-3720.

[15] Goette A, Honeycntt C, Langberg JJ: Electrical remoldeling in atrial fibrillation time course and mechanisms. Circulation 94: 2968,

1996.

[16] Wijffels MC, Kirchhof CJ, Dorland R, et al. Electrical remodeling due to atrial fibrillation in chronically instrumented conscious goats: roles of neurohumoral changes, ischemia, atrial stretch, and high rate of electrical activation [J]. Circulation, 1997, 96: 3710-3720.

[17] Ingemansson MP, Holm M, Olsson SB: Autonomic modulation of the atrial cycle length by the head up tilt test: non-invasive evaluation in patients with chronic atrial fibrillation. Heart, 1998, 80: 71-76.

[18] Elvan A, Wylie K, Zipes DP: Pacing-induced chronic atrial fibrillation impairs sinus node function in dogs. Electrophysiological remodeling. Circulation, 1996; 94, 2953-2960.

[19] Kanoupakis EM, Manios EG, Marrakis HE, Kaleboubas MD, Parthenakis FI: Relation of autonomic modulation to recurrence of atrial fibrillation following cardioversion. Am J Cardiol, 2000, 86: 954-958.

[20] Liu L, Nattel S. Differing sympathetic and vagal effects on atrial fibrillation in dogs: role of refractoriness heterogeneity [J]. Am J Physiol. 1997, 273: H805-816.

[21] Farch S, Villemaire C, Nattel S: Importance of refractoriness heterogeneity in the enhanced vulnerability to atrial fibrillation induction caused by tachycardia-induced atrial eletrical remodeling. Circulation, 1998, 98: 2202. Gaspo R, Bosch RF, Talajic M, et al. Functional mechanisms underlying tachycardia-induced sustained atrial fibrillation in a chronic dog model [J]. Circulation, 1997, 96: 4027-4035.

[22] Hirose M, Leatmanoratn Z, Laurita KR, et al. Effects of pituitary adenylate cyclase-activating polypeptide on canine atrial electrophysiology [J]. Am J Physiol Heart Circ Physiol, 2001, 281: H1667-1674.

[23] Farch S, Villemaire C, Nattel S. Importance of refractoriness heterogeneity in the enhanced vulnerability to atrial fibrillation induction caused by tachycardia-induced atrial electrical remodeling [J]. Circulation, 1998, 98: 2202-2209.

[24] Tieleman RG, Delangen C, Van Gelder IC: Regional differences in pacing induced electrical remodeling induces dispersion of refractoriness. Circulation, 1996, 94: I-352.

[25] Chen YJ, Tai CT, Chion CW, Wen ZC, Chan P, et al: Inducibillity of atrial fibrillation during atrioventricular pacing with varying intervals: role of atrial electrophysiology and the autonomic nervous system. J Cardiovasc Electrophysio, 1999, 10: 1578-1585.

[26] 唐丽萍, 庄亚纯, 刘忠豫, 等. 犬心率变异的实验研究. 中国心脏起搏与心电生理杂志, 1998, 12: 158-160.

第2章

[1] Huang CX, Zhao QY, Jiang H, et al. Experimental study of the effect of the vagus nerve on atrial electrical remodeling[J]. J of Electrocardiology, 2003, 36: 295.

[2] Schauerte P, Scherlag BJ, Patterson E, et al. Focal atrial fibrillation: Experimental evidence for a pathophysiologic role of the autonomic nervous system[J]. J Cardiovasc Electrophysiol, 2001, 12: 592.

[3] Pappone C, Santinelli V, Manguso F, et al. Pulmonary vein denervation enhances long-term benefit after circumferential ablation for paroxysmal atrial fibrillation[J]. Circulation, 2004, 109: 327.

[4] Nattel S. New ideas about atrial fibrillation 50 years on[J]. Nature, 2002, 415: 219.

[5] Chevalier P, Tabib A, Meyronnet D, Chalabreysse L, Restier L, Ludman V, Alies A, Adeleine P, Thivolet F, Burri H, Loire R, Francois L, Fanton L: Quantitative study of nerves of the human

left atrium. Heart Rhythm 2005, 2, 518-522.

[6] Zou R, Kneller J, Leon LJ, et al. Substrate size as a determinant of fibrillatory activity maintenance in a mathematical model of canine atrium. Am J Physiol Heart Circ Physiol, 2005, 289: 1002-1012.

[7] Chiou CW, Eble JN, Zipes DP. Efferent vagal innervation of the canine atria and sinus and atrioventricular nodes. The third fat pad. Circulation, 1997, 95: 2573-84.

[8] Sharifov OF, Fedorov VV, Beloshapko GG, et al. Roles of adrenergic and cholinergic stimulation in spontaneous atrial fibrillation in dogs. J Am Coll Cardiol, 2004, 43: 483-490.

[9] Po SS, Scherlag BJ, Yamanashi WS, et al. Experimental model for paroxysmal atrial fibrillation arising at the pulmonary vein-atrial junctions. Heart Rhythm. 2006, 3, 201-208.

[10] Kovoor P, Wickman K, Maguire CT, et al. Evaluation of the role of I_{KAch} in atrial fibrillation using a mouse knockout model[J]. J Am Coll Cardiol, 2001, 37: 2136.

[11] Mansour M, Mandapati R, Berenfeld O, et al. Left-to-right gradient of atrial frequencies during acute atrial fibrillation in the isolated sheep heart[J]. Circulation, 2001, 103: 2631.

[12] Wang YG, Huser J, Blatter LA, et al. Withdrawal of acetylcholine elicits Ca^{2+}-induced delayed after depolarizations in cat atrial myocytes[J]. Circulation, 1997, 96: 1275.

[13] Smeets JL, Allessie MA, Lammers WJ, Bonke FI, Hollen J: The wavelength of the cardiac impulse and reentrant arrhythmias in isolated rabbit atrium: The role of heart rate, autonomic transmitters, temperature, and potassium. Circ Res, 1986, 58: 96-108.

[14] Waldo AL: Mechanisms of atrial fibrillation. J Cardiovasc Electrophysiol, 2003, 14: S267-S274.

[15] Li D, Zhang L, Kneller J, Nattel S. Potential ionic mechanism for repolarization differences between canine right and left atrium[J].

Circulation Research, 2001, 88: 1168-1175.

[16] Schuessler RB, Grayson TM, Bromberg BI, et al. Cholinergically mediated tachyarrhythmias induced by a single extrastimulus in the isolated canine right atrium [J]. Circulation Research, 1992, 71: 1254-1267.

[17] Allessie MA, Lammers WJEP, Bonke FIM, et al. Experimental evaluation of Moe's multiple wavelet hypothesis of atrial fibrillation. In Zipes DP, Jalife J, eds: Cardiac Electrophysiology and Arrhythmias. Orlando, FL: Grune & Stratton, 1985, 265-276.

[18] Hirose M, Carlson MD, Laurita KR. Cellular mechanisms of vagally mediated atrial tachyarrhythmia in isolated arterially perfused canine right atria [J]. J Cardiovasc Electrophysiol, 2002, 13: 918.

[19] Watanabe Y, Hara Y, Tamagawa M, et al. Inhibitory effect of amiodarone on the muscarinic acetylcholine receptor-operated potassium current in guinea pig atrial cells. J Pharmacol Exp Ther. 1996, 279: 617-624.

[20] Varro A, Biliczki P, Iost N. et al. Theoretical possibilities for the development of novel antiarrhythmic drugs. Curr Med Chem. 2004, 11: 1-11.

第3章

[1] Huang CX, Zhao QY, Jiang H, et al. Experimental study of the effect of the vagus nerve on atrial electrical remodeling [J]. J of Electrocardiology, 2003, 36: 295.

[2] Schauerte P, Scherlag BJ, Patterson E, et al. Focal atrial fibrillation: Experimental evidence for a pathophysiologic role of the autonomic nervous system [J]. J Cardiovasc Electrophysiol, 2001, 12: 592.

[3] 赵庆彦, 黄从新, 杨波, 等. 迷走神经对心房有效不应期离散

度影响的实验研究 [J]. 中国循环杂志, 2003, 18: 221-223.

[4] Pappone C, Santinelli V, Manguso F, et al. Pulmonary vein denervation enhances long-term benefit after circumferential ablation for paroxysmal atrial fibrillation [J]. Circulation, 2004, 109: 327.

[5] Chiou CW, Eble JN, Zipes DP. Efferent vagal innervation of the canine atria and sinus and atrioventricular nodes. The third fat pad. Circulation [J]. 1997, 95: 2573-84.

[6] Scherlag BJ, Nakagawa H, Jackman WM, et al. Electrical stimulation to identify neural elements on the heart: their role in atrial fibrillation [J]. J Interv Card Electrophysiol, 2005, 13 Suppl 1: 37-42.

[7] Quan KJ, Lee JH, Geha AS, et al. Characterization of sinoatrial parasympathetic innervation in humans [J]. J Cardiovasc Electrophysiol, 1999, 10: 1060-1065.

[8] Quan KJ, Lee JH, Van Hare GF, et al. Identification and characterization of atrioventricular parasympathetic innervation in humans [J]. J Cardiovasc Electrophysiol, 2002, 13: 735-739.

[9] 黄从新, 谢强, 吴钢, 等. 犬 Marshall 韧带内心肌细胞短暂外向钾电流的特性. 中华心律失常学杂志, 2004, 4: 228-232.

[10] Shi H, Wang H, Wang Z: Identification and characterization of multiple subtypes of muscarinic acetylcholine receptors and their physiological functions in canine hearts. Mol Pharmacol, 1999, 55: 497-507.

[11] Mansour M, Mandapati R, Berenfeld O, et al. Left-to-right gradient of atrial frequencies during acute atrial fibrillation in the isolated sheep heart [J]. Circulation, 2001, 103: 2631.

[12] Hirose M, Carlson MD, Laurita KR. Cellular mechanisms of vagally mediated atrial tachyarrhythmia in isolated arterially perfused canine right atria [J]. J Cardiovasc Electrophysiol, 2002, 13: 918.

[13] Sarmast F, Kolli A, Zaitsev A, et al. Cholinergic atrial fibrilla-

tion: I_{KAch} gradients determine unequal left/right atrial frequencies and rotor dynamics. Cardiovasc Res, 2003, 59: 863-873.

[14] Lomax AE, Kondo CS, Giles WR, et al. Comparison of time-and voltage-dependent K^+ currents in myocytes from left and right atria of adult mice[J]. Am J Physiol Heart Circ Physiol, 2003, 285: H1837

[15] Lomax AE, Rose RA, Giles WR. et al. Electrophysiological evidence for a gradient of G protein-gated K^+ current in adult mouse atria[J]. Br J Pharmacol, 2003, 140: 576.

[16] Bettoni M, Zimmermann M. Autonomic tone variations before the onset of paroxysmal atrial fibrillation [J]. Circulation, 2002, 105: 2753-2759.

[17] Oral H, Chugh A, Scharf C, Hall B, Cheung P, Veerareddy S, Daneshvar GF, Pelosi F Jr, Morady F. Pulmonary vein isolation for vagotonic, adrenergic, and random episodes of paroxysmal atrial fibrillation. J Cardiovasc Electrophysiol, 2004, 15: 402-406.

[18] Razavi M, Zhang S, Yang D, et al. Effects of pulmonary vein ablation on regional atrial vagal innervation and vulnerability to atrial fibrillation in dogs. J Cardiovasc Electrophysiol, 2005, 16: 879-884.

[19] Yamada M, Inanobe A, Kurachi Y, et al. G protein regulation of potassium ion channels[J]. Pharmacol Rev, 1998, 50: 723.

[20] Krapivinsky G, Gordon EA, Wickman K, et al. The G-protein-gated atrial K^+ channel IKAch is a heteromultimer of two inwardly rectifying K^+-channel proteins[J]. Nature, 1995, 374: 135

[21] Bettahi I, Marker CL, Roman MI, et al. Contribution of the Kir3.1 subunit to the muscarinic-gated atrial potassium channel IKAch [J]. Biol Chem, 2002, 13: 48282.

[22] Logothetis DE, Kurachi Y, Galper J, et al. The beta gamma subunits of GTP-binding proteins activate the muscarinic K^+ channel in heart[J]. Nature, 1987, 325: 321.

[23] Sharifov OF, Zaitsev AV, Rosenshtraukh LV, et al. Spatial distribution and frequency-dependence of arrhythmogenic vagal effects in canine atria. J Cardiovasc Electrophysiol, 2000, 11: 1029-1042.

[24] Watanabe Y, Hara Y, Tamagawa M, et al. Inhibitory effect of amiodarone on the muscarinic acetylcholine receptor-operated potassium current in guinea pig atrial cells. J Pharmacol Exp Ther, 1996, 279: 617-624.

[25] Brandts B, Borchard R, Macianskiene R, et al. Inhibition of G protein-coupled and ATP-sensitive potassium currents by 2-methyl-3-(3, 5-diiodo- 4-carboxymethoxybenzyl) benzofuran (KB130015), an amiodarone derivative. J Pharmacol Exp Ther, 2004, 308: 134-142.

[26] Borchard R, van Bracht M, Wickenbrock I, et al. Inhibition of the muscarinic potassium current by KB130015, a new antiarrhythmic agent to treat atrial fibrillation. Med Klin, 2005, 100: 697-703.

第4章

[1] Van Wagoner DR, N erbonne JM. Molecular basis of electrical remodeling in atrial fibrillation [J]. J Mol Cell Cardiol. 2000, 32: 1101-17.

[2] Huang CX, Zhao QY, Jiang H, et al. Experimental study of the effect of the vagus nerve on atrial electrical remodeling [J]. J of Electrocardiology, 2003, 36: 295.

[3] Schauerte P, Scherlag BJ, Patterson E, et al. Focal atrial fibrillation: Experimental evidence for a pathophysiologic role of the autonomic nervous system [J]. J Cardiovasc Electrophysiol, 2001, 12: 592-599.

[4] 赵庆彦, 黄从新, 杨波, 等. 迷走神经对心房有效不应期离散度影响的实验研究 [J]. 中国循环杂志, 2003, 18: 221-223.

[5] Pappone C, Santinelli V, Manguso F, et al. Pulmonary vein denervation enhances long-term benefit after circumferential ablation for

paroxysmal atrial fibrillation [J]. Circulation, 2004, 109: 327-334.

[6] Randall WC, Ardell JL. Selective parasympathectomy of automatic and conductile tissues of the canine heart. Am J Physiol, 1985, 248: H61-H68.

[7] Randall WC, Ardell JL, O'Toole MF, et al. Differential autonomic control of SAN and AVN regions of the canine heart: Structure and function. Prog Clin Biol Res, 1998, 275: 15-31.

[8] Billman GE, Hoskins RS, Randall DC, et al. Selective vagal postganglionic innervation of the sinoatrial and atrioventricular nodes in the non-human primate. J Auton Nerv Syst, 1989, 26: 27-36.

[9] Chiou CW, Eble JN, Zipes DP. Efferent vagal innervation of the canine atria and sinus and atrioventricular nodes. The third fat pad. Circulation[J], 1997, 95: 2573-2584.

[10] Scherlag BJ, Nakagawa H, Jackman WM, et al. Electrical stimulation to identify neural elements on the heart: their role in atrial fibrillation[J]. J Interv Card Electrophysiol, 2005, 13 Suppl 1: 37-42.

[11] Quan KJ, Lee JH, Geha AS, et al. Characterization of sinoatrial parasympathetic innervation in humans [J]. J Cardiovasc Electrophysiol, 1999, 10: 1060-1065.

[12] Quan KJ, Lee JH, Van Hare GF, et al. Identification and characterization of atrioventricular parasympathetic innervation in humans [J]. J Cardiovasc Electrophysiol, 2002, 13: 735-739.

[13] Chevalier P, Tabib A, Meyronnet D, et al. Quantitative study of nerves of the human left atrium. Heart Rhythm[J]. 2005; 2: 518-22.

[14] El-Sherif N. Paroxysmal atrial flutter and fibrillation. Induction by carotid sinus compression and prevention by atropine [J]. Br Heart J, 1972, 34: 1024-1028.

[15] Wilson CL, Davis SJ. Recurrent atrial fibrillation with nausea and

vomiting [J]. Aviat Space Environ Med, 1978, 49: 624-625.

[16] Coumel P, Attuel P, Lavallee J, et al. The atrial arrhythmia syndrome of vagal origin [J]. Arch Mal Coeur Vaiss, 1978, 71: 645-56.

[17] Coumel P. Autonomic influences in atrial tachyarrhythmias. J Cardiovasc Electrophysiol, 1996, 7: 999-1007.

[18] Chen YJ, Chen SA, Tai CT, Wen ZC, Feng AN, Ding YA, Chang MS: Role of atrial electrophysiology and autonomic nervous system in patients with supraventricular tachycardia and paroxysmal atrial fibrillation. J Am Coll Cardiol, 1998, 32: 732-738.

[19] Singh J, Mela T, Ruskin J. Sleep (vagal)-induced atrial fibrillation. Circulation, 2004, 110: 32-33.

[20] Bettoni M, Zimmermann M. Autonomic tone variations before the onset of paroxysmal atrial fibrillation [J]. Circulation, 2002, 105: 2753-2759.

[21] Fioranelli M, Piccoli M, Mileto GM, et al. Analysis of heart rate variability five minutes before the onset of paroxysmal atrial fibrillation [J]. PACE, 1999, 22: 743-749.

[22] Tomita T, Takei M, Saikawa Y, et al. Role of autonomic tone in the initiation and termination of paroxysmal atrial fibrillation in patients without structural heart disease. J Cardiovasc Electrophysiol, 2003, 14: 565-566.

[23] Bertaglia E, Zoppo F, Bonanno C, et al. Autonomic modulation of the sinus node following electrical cardioversion of persistent atrial fibrillation: relation with early recurrence. In J Cardiol, 2005, 102: 219-23.

[24] Vikman S, Makikallio TH, Yli-Mayry S, et al. Heart rate variability and recurrence of atrial fibrillation after electrical cardioversion. Ann Med, 2003, 35: 36-42.

[25] Vikman S, Lindgren K, Makikallio TH, et al. Heart rate turbulence after atrial premature beats before spontaneous onset of atrial

fibrillation. J Am Coll Cardiol, 2005, 45: 278-284.

[26] Sutton AG, Khurana C, Hall JA, et al. The use of atropine for facilitation of direct current cardioversion from atrial fibrillation--results of a pilot study[J]. Clin Cardiol, 1999, 22: 712-714.

[27] Scherlag BJ, Yamanashi W, Patel U, et al. Autonomically induced conversion of pulmonary vein focal firing into atrial fibrillation[J]. J Am Coll Cardiol, 2005, 45: 1878-1886.

[28] Wang J, Liu L, Feng J, et al. Regional and functional factors determining induction and maintenance of atrial fibrillation in dogs [J]. Am J Physiol, 1996, 271: H148-H158.

[29] Schauerte P, Scherlag BJ, Patterson E, et al. Focal atrial fibrillation: experimental evidence for a pathophysiologic role of the autonomic nervous system[J]. J Cardiovasc Electrophysiol, 2001, 12: 592-599.

[30] Sharifov OF, Fedorov VV, Beloshapko GG, et al. Roles of adrenergic and cholinergic stimulation in spontaneous atrial fibrillation in dogs. J Am Coll Cardiol, 2004, 43: 483-490.

[31] Po SS, Scherlag BJ, Yamanashi WS, et al. Experimental model for paroxysmal atrial fibrillation arising at the pulmonary vein-atrial junctions. Heart RHYthm, 2006, 3: 201-208.

[32] Akyurek O, Diker E, Guldal M, et al. Predictive value of heart rate variability for the recurrence of chronic atrial fibrillation after electrical cardioversion. Clin Cardiol, 2003, 26: 196-200.

[33] Lombardi F, Tarricone D, Tundo F, et al. Autonomic nervous system and paroxysmal atrial fibrillation: a study based on the analysis of RR interval changes before, during and after paroxysmal atrial fibrillation. Eur Heart J, 2004, 25: 1242-1248.

[34] van den Berg MP, Hassink RJ, Balje-Volkers C, et al. Role of the autonomic nervous system in vagal atrial fibrillation. Heart, 2003, 89: 333-335.

[35] Kanoupakis EM, Manios EG, Mavrakis HE, et al. Relation of au-

tonomic modulation to recurrence of atrial fibrillation following cardioversion [J]. Am J Cardiol, 2000, 86: 954-958.

[36] Alessi R, Nusynowitz M, Abildskov JA, et al. Nonuniform distribution of vagal effects on the atrial refractory period. Am J Physiol, 1958, 194: 406-410.

[37] Zipes DP, Mihalick MJ, Robbins GT. Effects of selective vagal and stellate ganglion stimulation on atrial refractoriness. Circ Res, 1974, 8: 647-655.

[38] Liu L, Nattel S. Differing sympathetic and vagal effects on atrial fibrillation in dogs: role of refractoriness heterogeneity. Am J Physiol, 1997, 273: H805-H816.

[39] Jalife J, Berenfeld O, Skanes A. et al. Mechanisms of atrial fibrillation: mother rotors or multiple daughter wavelets, or both[J]? J Cardiovasc Electrophysiol, 1998, 9: S2-S12.

[40] Sharifov OF, Zaitsev AV, Rosenshtraukh LV, et al. Spatial distribution and frequency dependence of arrhythmogenic vagal effects in canine atria[J]. J Cardiovasc Electrophysiol, 2000, 11: 1029-1042.

[41] Schauerte P, Scherlag BJ, Pitha J, et al. Catheter ablation of cardiac autonomic nerves for prevention of vagal atrial fibrillation[J]. Circulation, 2000, 102: 2774-2780.

[42] Goette A, Honeycutt C, Langberg JJ. Electrical remodeling in atrial fibrillation. Time course and mechanisms[J]. Circulation, 1996, 94: 2968-2974.

[43] Takei M, Tsuboi M, Usui T, et al. Vagal stimulation prior to atrial rapid pacing protects the atrium from electrical remodeling in anesthetized dogs[J]. Jpn Circ J, 2001, 65: 1077-1081.

[44] Blaauw Y, Tieleman RG, BrouwerJ, et al. Tachycardia induced electrical remodeling of the atria and the autonomic nervous system in goats[J]. PACE, 1999, 22: 1656-1667.

[45] Miyauchi M, Kobayashi Y, MiyauchiY, et al. Parasympathetic

blockade promotes recovery from atrial electrical remodeling induced by short-term rapid atrial pacing. PACE, 2004 Jan, 27 (1): 33-37.

[46] Wijffels MC, Kirchhof CJ, Dorland R, et al. Electrical remodeling due to atrial fibrillation in chronically instrumented conscious goats: roles of neurohumoral changes, ischemia, atrial stretch, and high rate of electrical activation[J]. Circulation, 1997, 96: 3710-3720.

[47] Tieleman RG, Blaauw Y, Van Gelder IC, et al. Digoxin delays recovery from tachycardia-induced electrical remodeling of the atria [J]. Circulation, 1999, 26; 100: 1836-1842.

[48] Gaspo R, Bosch RF, Talajic M, et al. Functional mechanisms underlying tachycardia-induced sustained atrial fibrillation in a chronic dog model[J]. Circulation, 1997, 96: 4027-4035.

[49] Liu L, Nattel S. Differing sympathetic and vagal effects on atrial fibrillation in dogs: role of refractoriness heterogeneity[J]. Am J Physiol, 1997, 273: H805-816.

[50] Hirose M, Leatmanoratn Z, Laurita KR, et al. Effects of pituitary adenylate cyclase-activating polypeptide on canine atrial electrophysiology[J]. Am J Physiol Heart Circ Physiol, 2001, 281: H1667-1674.

[51] Chen YJ, Chen SA, Tai CT, et al. Role of atrial electrophysiology and autonomic nervous system in patients with supraventricular tachycardia and paroxyamal atrial fibrillation [J]. J Am Coll Cardiol, 1998, 32: 732.

[52] Chen YJ, Tai CT, Chiou CW, et al. Indecibillity of atrial fibrillation during atrioventricular pacing with varying intervals: role of atrial electrophysiology and the autonomic nervous system [J]. J cardiovasc Electrophysiol, 1999, 10: 1578-1585.

[53] Farch S, Villemaire C, Nattel S. Importance of refractoriness heterogeneity in the enhanced vulnerability to atrial fibrillation induction

caused by tachycardia-induced atrial electrical remodeling [J]. Circulation, 1998, 98: 2202-2209.

[54] Smeets JL, Allessie MA, Lammers WJ, Bonke FI, Hollen J. The wavelength of the cardiac impulse and reentrant arrhythmias in isolated rabbit atrium: The role of heart rate, autonomic transmitters, temperature, and potassium. Circ Res, 1986, 58: 96-108.

[55] Waldo AL. Mechanisms of atrial fibrillation. J Cardiovasc Electrophysiol, 2003, 14: S267-S274.

[56] Li D, Zhang L, Kneller J, Nattel S. Potential ionic mechanism for repolarization differences between canine right and left atrium[J]. Circulation Research, 2001, 88: 1168-1175.

[57] Schuessler RB, Grayson TM, Bromberg BI, Cox JL, Boineau JP. Cholinergically mediated tachyarrhythmias induced by a single extrastimulus in the isolated canine right atrium[J]. Circulation Research, 1992, 71: 1254-1267.

[58] Allessie MA, Lammers WJEP, Bonke FIM, Hollen J. Experimental evaluation of Moe's multiple wavelet hypothesis of atrial fibrillation. In Zipes DP, Jalife J, eds. Cardiac Electrophysiology and Arrhythmias. Orlando, FL: Grune & Stratton, 1985, 265-276.

[59] Hirose M, Carlson MD, Laurita KR. Cellular mechanisms of vagally mediated atrial tachyarrhythmia in isolated arterially perfused canine right atria [J]. J Cardiovasc Electrophysiol, 2002, 13: 918.

[60] Ashihara T, Yao T, Namba T, et al. Differences in sympathetic and vagal effects on paroxysmal atrial fibrillation: A simulation study[J]. Biomed Pharmacother, 2002, 56 Suppl 2: 359.

[61] Vigmond EJ, Tsoi V, KuoS, et al. The effect of vagally induced dispersion of action potential duration on atrial arrhythmogenesis. Heart Rhythm, 2004, 1: 334-344.

[62] 赵庆彦，黄从新，梁锦军，等．迷走神经刺激及I_{KAch}在犬心房的分布特点对心房颤动影响的机制研究．中华心血管杂志，

2006, 4: 48-49.

[63] Liu L, Nattel. S. Differing sympathetic and vagal effects on atrial fibrillation in dogs: role of refractoriness heterogeneity[J]. Am J Physiol, 1997, 273: H805-H16.

[64] Olgin JE, Sih HJ, Hanish S, et al. Heterogeneous atrial denervation creates substrate for sustained atrial fibrillation[J]. Circulation, 1998, 98: 2608-2614.

[65] Patterson E, Po SS, Scherlag BJ, et al. Triggered firing in pulmonary veins initiated by in vitro autonomic nerve stimulation[J]. Heart Rhythm, 2005, 2: 624-631.

[66] Hara Y, Nakaya H. Dual effects of extracellular ATP on the muscarinic acetylcholine receptor-operated K^+ current in guinea-pig atrial cells[J]. Eur J Pharmacol, 1997, 324: 295.

[67] Kurachi Y, Ishii M: Cell signal control of the G protein-gated potassium channel and its subcellular localization. J Physiol, 2004, 554: 285-294.

[68] Wang Z, Shi H, Wang H. Functional M3 muscarinic acetylcholine receptors in mammalian hearts[J]. Br J Pharmacol, 2004, 142: 395-408.

[69] Shi H, Wang H, Yang B, et al. The M3 receptor-mediated K^+ current (IKM3), a G(q) protein-coupled K^+ channel[J]. J Biol Chem, 2004, 279: 21774-21778.

[70] Shi H, Yang B, Xu D, et al. Electrophysiological characterization of cardiac muscarinic acetylcholine receptors: different subtypes mediate different potassium currents[J]. Cell Physiol Biochem, 2003, 13: 59-74.

[71] Yamada M, Inanobe A, Kurachi Y, et al. G protein regulation of potassium ion channels[J]. Pharmacol Rev, 1998, 50: 723.

[72] Krapivinsky G, Gordon EA, Wickman K, et al. The G-protein-gated atrial K^+ channel IKAch is a heteromultimer of two inwardly rectifying K^+-channel proteins[J]. Nature, 1995, 374: 135.

[73] Bettahi I, Marker CL, Roman MI, et al. Contribution of the Kir3.1 subunit to the muscarinic-gated atrial potassium channel IKAch [J]. Biol Chem, 2002, 13: 48282

[74] Logothetis DE, Kurachi Y, Galper J, et al. The beta gamma subunits of GTP-binding proteins activate the muscarinic K$^+$ channel in heart[J]. Nature, 1987, 325: 321.

[75] Bettahi I, Marker CL, Roman MI, et al. Contribution of the Kir3.1 subunit to the muscarinic-gated atrial potassium channel IKAch [J]. J Biol Chem, 2002, 277: 48, 282.

[76] Sarmast F, Kolli A, Zaitsev A, et al. Cholinergic atrial fibrillation: I_{KAch} gradients determine unequal left/right atrial frequencies and rotor dynamics[J]. Cardiovasc Res, 2003, 59: 863.

[77] Lomax AE, Kondo CS, Giles WR. et al. Comparison of time-and voltage-dependent K$^+$ currents in myocytes from left and right atria of adult mice[J]. Am J Physiol Heart Circ Physiol, 2003, 285: H1837.

[78] Lomax AE, Rose RA, Giles WR. et al. Electrophysiological evidence for a gradient of G protein-gated K$^+$ current in adult mouse atria[J]. Br J Pharmacol, 2003, 140: 576.

[79] Huang congxin, Zhao Qingyan, Liang Jinjun, et al. Differential densities of Muscarinic acetylcholone receptor and $I_{K,Ach}$ in canine supraventricular tissues and the effect of amiodarone on cholinergical atrial fibrillation and $I_{K,Ach}$[J]. Cardiology, 2006, 106: 36-43.

[80] Kovoor P, Wickman K, Maguire CT, et al. Evaluation of the role of I_{KAch} in atrial fibrillation using a mouse knockout model[J]. J Am Coll Cardiol, 2001, 37: 2136.

[81] Mansour M, Mandapati R, Berenfeld O, et al. Left-to-right gradient of atrial frequencies during acute atrial fibrillation in the isolated sheep heart[J]. Circulation, 2001, 103: 2631.

[82] Li D, Zhang L, Kneller J, et al. Potential ionic mechanism for re-

polarization differences between canine right and left atrium[J]. Circ Res, 2001, 88: 1168.

[83] Nattel S. New ideas about atrial fibrillation 50 years on[J]. Nature, 2002, 415: 219

[84] Chevalier P, Tabib A, Meyronnet D, Chalabreysse L, Restier L, Ludman V, Alies A, Adeleine P, Thivolet F, Burri H, Loire R, Francois L, Fanton L: Quantitative study of nerves of the human left atrium. Heart Rhythm, 2005, 2: 518-522.

[85] Zou R, Kneller J, Leon LJ, et al. Substrate size as a determinant of fibrillatory activity maintenance in a mathematical model of canine atrium. Am J Physiol Heart Circ Physiol, 2005, 289: 1002-1012.

[86] Wang YG, Huser J, Blatter LA, et al. Withdrawal of acetylcholine elicits Ca^{2+}-induced delayed afterdepolarizations in cat atrial myocytes[J]. Circulation, 1997, 96: 1275.

[87] Shi H, Wang H, Li D, et al. Differential alterations of receptor densities of three muscarinic acetylcholine receptor subtypes and current densities of the corresponding K^+ channels in canine atria with atrial fibrillation induced by experimental congestive heart failure[J]. Cell Physiol Biochem, 2004, 14: 31.

[88] Dobrev D, Graf E, Wettwer E, et al. Molecular basis of downregulation of G-protein-coupled inward rectifying K(+) current I_{KAch} in chronic human atrial fibrillation: decrease in GIRK4 mRNA correlates with reduced I_{KAch} and muscarinic receptor-mediated shortening of action potentials[J]. Circulation, 2001, 104: 2551.

[89] Dobrev D, Friedrich A, Voigt N, et al. The G protein-gated potassium current I(K, Ach) is constitutively active in patients with chronic atrial fibrillation. Circulation, 2005, 112: 3697-3706.

[90] Watanabe Y, Hara Y, Tamagawa M, et al. Inhibitory effect of amiodarone on the muscarinic acetylcholine receptor-operated potassium current in guinea pig atrial cells. J Pharmacol Exp Ther, 1996,

279: 617-624.

[91] Varro A, Biliczki P, Iost N. et al. Theoretical possibilities for the development of novel antiarrhythmic drugs. Curr Med Chem, 2004, 11: 1-11.

[92] Brandts B, Borchard R, Macianskiene R, Gendviliene V, Dirkmann D, Van Bracht M, Prull M, Meine M, Wickenbrock I, Mubagwa K, Trappe HJ. Inhibition of G protein-coupled and ATP-sensitive potassium currents by 2-methyl-3-(3, 5-diiodo- 4-carboxymethoxybenzyl) benzofuran (KB130015), an amiodarone derivative. J Pharmacol Exp Ther, 2004, 308: 134-142.

[93] Guillemare E, Marion A, Nisato D, et al. Inhibitory effects of dronedarone on muscarinic K^+ current in guinea pig atrial cells [J]. J Cardiovasc Pharmacol, 2000, 36: 802.

[94] Borchard R, van Bracht M, Wickenbrock I, et al. Inhibition of the muscarinic potassium current by KB130015, a new antiarrhythmic agent to treat atrial fibrillation. Med Klin, 2005, 100: 697-703.

[95] Watanabe Y, Hara Y, Tamagawa M, et al. Pirmenol inhibits muscarinic acetylcholine receptor-operated K^+ current in the guinea pig heart[J]. Eur J Pharmacol, 1997, 338: 71.

[96] Sugiura H, Chinushi M, Komura S, et al. Heart rate variability is a useful parameter for evaluation of anticholinergic effect associated with inducibility of atrial fibrillation. PACE, 2005, 28: 1208-1214.

[97] Fedorov VV, Rozenshtraukh LV, Reznik AV, et al. Antiarrhythmic Efficacy of a New Class III Antiarrhythmic Drug RG-2. Kardiologiia, 2004, 44: 66-73.

[98] Hara Y, Kizaki K. Antimalarial drugs inhibit the acetylcholine-receptor-operated potassium current in atrial myocytes. Heart Lung Circ, 2002, 11: 112-116.

[99] Randall WC, Kaye MP, Thomas JX Jr, et al. Intrapericardial denervation of the heart. J Surg Res, 1980, 29: 101.

[100] Randall WC, Thomas JX, Barber MJ, et al. Selective denervation of the heart. Am J Physiol, 1983, 244: H607-H613.

[101] Elvan A, Pride HP, Fble JN, et al. Radiofrequency catheter ablation of the atria reduces inducibility and duration of atrial fibrillation in dogs. Circulation, 1995, 91: 2235-2244.

[102] Hirose M, Leatmanoratn Z, Laurita KR, et al. Partial vagal denervation increases vulnerability to vagally induced atrial fibrillation. J Cardiovasc Electrophysiol, 2002, 13: 1272-1279.

[103] Nakagawa H, Scherlag BJ, Aoyamo H, et al. Catherter ablation of cardiac autonomic nerves for prevention of atrial fibrillation in a canine model. Heart Rhythm, 2004, 1: S10.

[104] Razavi M, Zhang S, Yang D, Sanders RA, Kar B, Delapasse S, Ai T, Moreira W, Olivier B, Khoury DS, Cheng J. Effects of pulmonary vein ablation on regional atrial vagal innervation and vulnerability to atrial fibrillation in dogs. J Cardiovasc Electrophysiol, 2005, 16: 879-884.

[105] Platt M, Mandapati R, Scherlag BJ, et al. Limiting the number and extent of radiofrequency applications to terminate atrial fibrillation and eubsequently prevent its inducibility. Heart Rhythm, 2004, 1: S11.

[106] Pappone C, Santinelli V. Atrial Fibrillation Ablation: State of the Art. Am J Cardiol, 2005, 96: 59-64.

[107] Takahashi Y, Jais P, Hocini M, et al. Shortening of fibrillatory cycle length in the pulmonary vein during vagal excitation. J Am Coll Cardiol, 2006, 47: 774-80.

[108] Oral H, Chugh A, Scharf C, et al. Pulmonary vein isolation for vagotonic, adrenergic, and random episodes of paroxysmal atrial fibrillation. J Cardiovasc Electrophysiol, 2004, 15: 402-406.

[109] Kocivic DZ, Harada T, Shea JB, et al. Alterations of heart rate and of heart rate variability after radiofrequency catheter ablation of supraventricular tachycardia. Delineation of parasympathetic

pathways in the human heart. Circulation, 1993, 88: 1671-1681.

[110] Chiou CW, Zipes DP. Selective vagal denervation of the atria eliminates heart rate variability and baroreflex sensitivity while preserving ventricular innervation. Circulation, 1998, 98: 360-368.

[111] Randall WC, Ardell JL: Selective parasympathectomy of automatic and conductile tissues of the canine heart. Am J Physiol, 1985, 248: H61-H68.

[112] Randall WC, Ardell JL, O'Toole MF, Wurster RD: Differential autonomic control of SAN and AVN regions of the canine heart: Structure and function. Prog Clin Biol Res, 1998, 275: 15-31.

[113] Billman GE, Hoskins RS, Randall DC, Randall WC, Hamlin RL, Lin YC: Selective vagal postganglionic innervation of the sinoatrial and atrioventricular nodes in the non-human primate. J Auton Nerv Syst, 1989, 26: 27-36.

[114] Cummings JE, Gill I, Akhrass R, Dery M, Biblo LA, Quan KJ: Preservation of the anterior fat pad paradoxically decreases the incidence of postoperative atrial fibrillation in humans. J Am Coll Cardiol, 2004, 43: 994-1000.

[115] Okuyama Y, Pak HN, Miyauchi Y, Liu YB, Chou CC, Hayashi H, Fu KJ, Kerwin WF, Kar S, Hata C, Karagueuzian HS, Fishbein MC, Chen PS, Chen LS: Nerve sprouting induced by radio-frequency catheter ablation in dogs. Heart Rhythm, 2004, 1: 712-717.

[116] Hamabe A, Chang CM, Zhou SM, Chou CC, Yi J, Miyauchi Y, Okuyama Y, Fishbein MC, Karagueuzian HS, Chen LS, Chen PS: Induction of atrial fibrillation and nerve sprouting by prolonged left atrial pacing in dogs. Pacing Clin Electrophysiol, 2003, 26: 2247-2252.

[117] Quan KJ, Lee JH, Van Hare GF, Biblo LA, Mackall JA, Carl-

son MD: Identification and characterization of atrioventricular parasympathetic innervation in humans. J Cardiovasc Electrophysiol, 2002, 13: 735-739.

后　记

　　衷心感谢导师黄从新教授在我攻读学位期间对我的辛勤培养和悉心指导，他渊博的知识、严谨求实的治学态度，对事业无私奉献的精神，以及在科研和行政管理上所体现出来的睿智和远见将影响我一生，并激励我在今后的工作和学习中不断进取和提高！

　　衷心感谢李庚山教授、唐其柱教授、江洪教授、杨波教授等各位老师的帮助，他们多年来的鼓励和教诲是我不断进取的动力！

　　衷心感谢唐艳红老师、王腾老师、胡萍老师等位老师和同学所给予的帮助，使我的学习生活变得紧张而富有成效！

　　衷心感谢林青老师、徐丽娟老师、刘志勇老师在校期间的关怀和培养！

　　衷心感谢我的家人及朋友多年来的一贯支持和帮助，他们的支持是我学业得以继续的保证！

武汉大学优秀博士学位论文文库

已出版：

- 基于双耳线索的移动音频编码研究／陈水仙　著
- 多帧影像超分辨率复原重建关键技术研究／谢伟　著
- Copula函数理论在多变量水文分析计算中的应用研究／陈璐　著
- 大型地下洞室群地震响应与结构面控制型围岩稳定研究／张雨霆　著
- 迷走神经诱发心房颤动的电生理和离子通道基础研究／赵庆彦　著
- 心房颤动的自主神经机制研究／鲁志兵　著
- 氧化应激状态下维持黑素小体蛋白低免疫原性的分子机制研究／刘小明　著
- 实流形在复流形中的全纯不变量／尹万科　著
- MITA介导的细胞抗病毒反应信号转导及其调节机制／钟波　著
- 图书馆数字资源选择标准研究／唐琼　著
- 年龄结构变动与经济增长：理论模型与政策建议／李魁　著
- 积极一般预防理论研究／陈金林　著
- 海洋石油开发环境污染法律救济机制研究／高翔　著
  ——以美国墨西哥湾漏油事故和我国渤海湾漏油事故为视角
- 中国共产党人政治忠诚观研究／徐霞　著
- 现代汉语属性名词语义特征研究／许艳平　著
- 论马克思的时间概念／熊进　著
- 晚明江南诗学研究／张清河　著